派螂蟷家朱

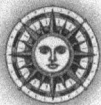

CHU GAR FIST
Hakka Southern Praying Mantis

Lao Sui's
Transmission to
Chu Kai Ming

SOM BO GIN SINGLE MAN

Three Step Arrow Form

Although, Southern Praying Mantis clans all share mostly the same basic skills, the Som Bo Gin form may vary to a greater degree from one to another. The common denominator is the three steps forward - three arrow punching followed by finger tip strikes.

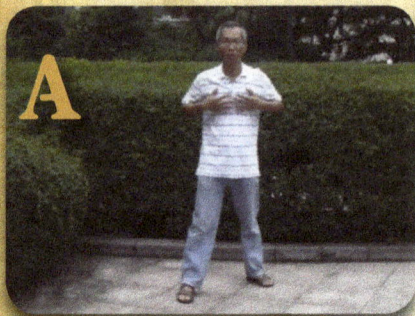

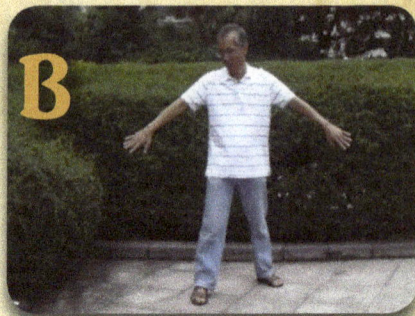

This "Som Bo Gin" form, in Southern Mantis, is written, in Chinese, by three different names: "Three Step Arrow" in Chu Gar, "Three Steps Forward" in Lam's USA Kwongsai Mantis, and "Three Steps Scissors" in China's Kwongsai Mantis.

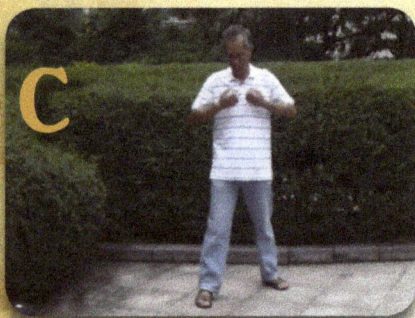

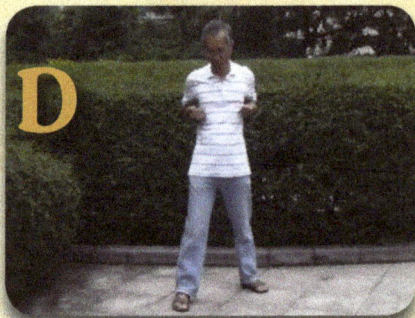

Read further, inside this book, about the form pictured here. And use the link below to garner detailed information about both Som Bo Gin Single Man and Two Man forms.

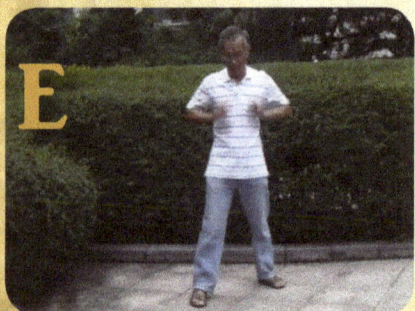

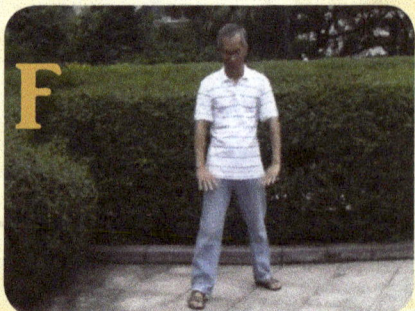

LINK TO SOM BO GIN TWO MAN FORM

southernmantispress.com/southern-praying-mantis-book-005.htm

三步進套路　HARD BRIDGE

Refer to Page 24

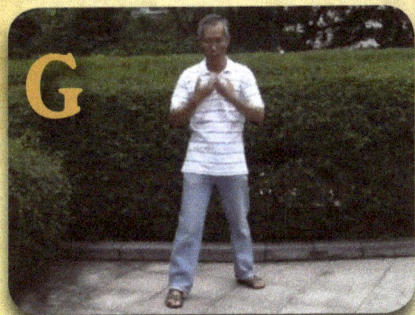

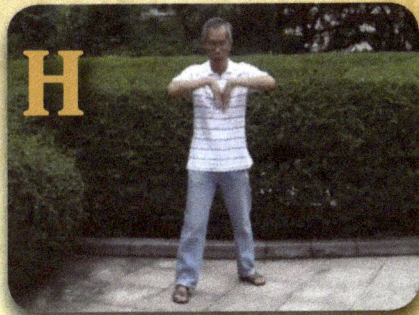

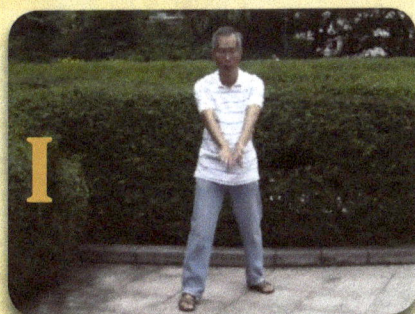

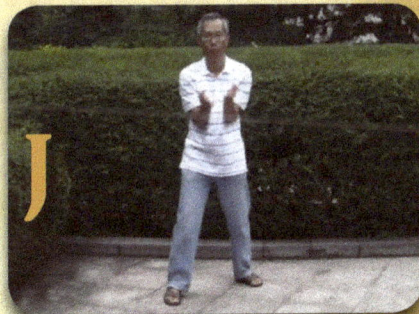

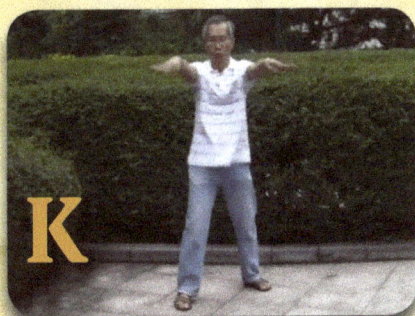

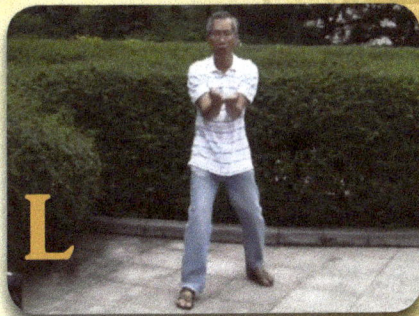

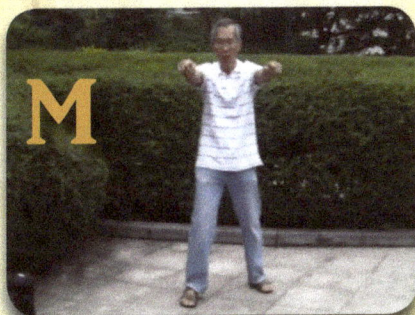

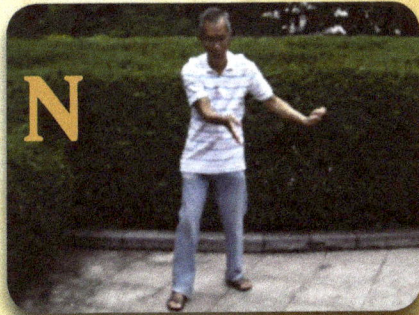

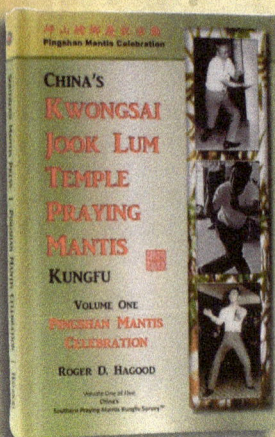

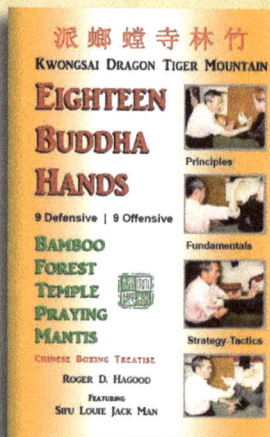

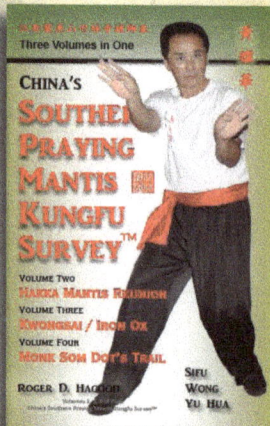

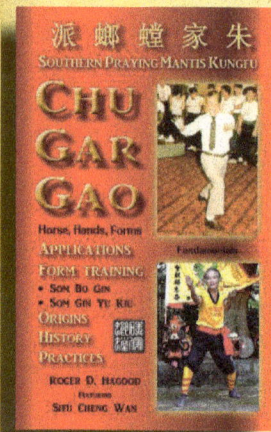

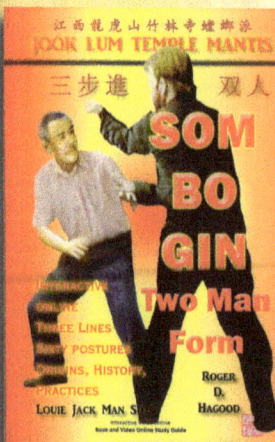

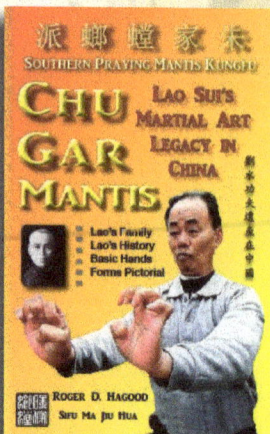

派 螂 螳 家 朱

Chu Gar Mantis

Lao Sui's Transmission to Chu Kai Ming

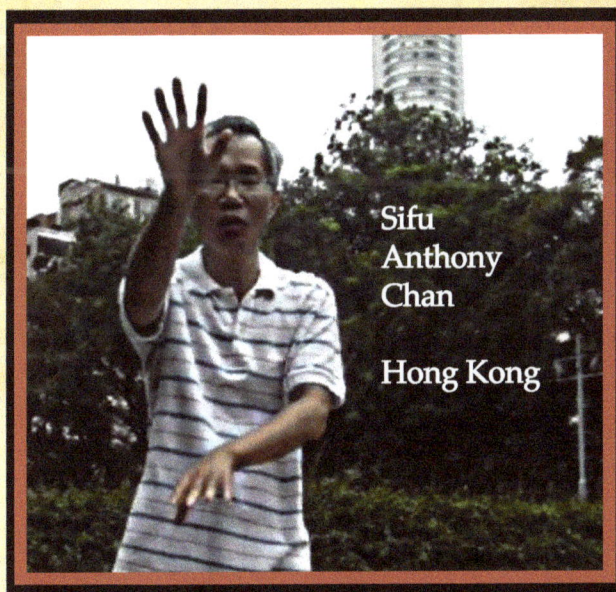

Sifu
Anthony
Chan

Hong Kong

By

Roger D. Hagood

Featuring
Sifu Anthony Chan

Editors
Charles Alan Clemens, Sean W. Robinson, Huang Yan

Southern Mantis Press | Pingshan Town, China

Southern Mantis Press
5424 NW Cascade Court
Camas, Washington, 98607
books@southernmantispress.com

Ordering Information:
Special discounts are available for martial art schools, bookstores, specialty shops, museums and events.   Contact the publisher at the address above.

Cover, Title Page, and Interior photographs: Sifu Anthony Chan, Hong Kong, Connoisseur of Hakka Southern Praying Mantis.

The cover image and all images in this book, of Chan Sifu, are captured from a consumer video camera recording. It was not originally intended for publication. Since recording, in 2013, we have decided to release this for preservation, promotion, and posterity of Hakka Mantis Kungfu.

ISBN: 978-0-9857240-8-5

Dedication

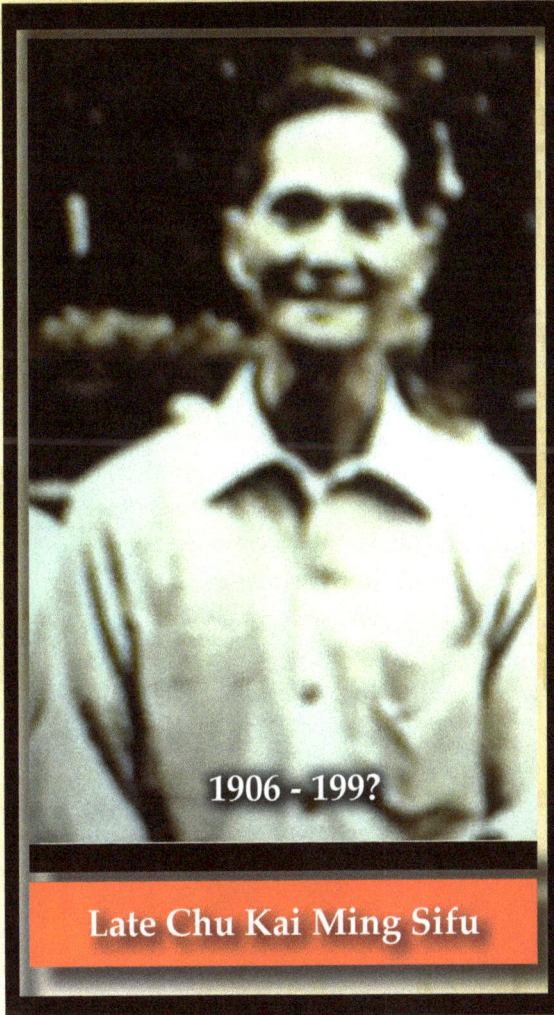

1906 - 199?

Late Chu Kai Ming Sifu

Anthony Chan Sifu is one of kind. To understand, you have to know him. The problem is he doesn't want to be known, by anyone. He is a Sifu, Historian, and Collector, of all things Hakka Kungfu, and especially Hakka Mantis, and that includes form and function of every Hakka boxing style, and he can play them all. His transmission is first generation Lao Sui Chu Gar Mantis from Chu Kai Ming, circa 1920s, Hong Kong.

Acknowledgement 拜人為師

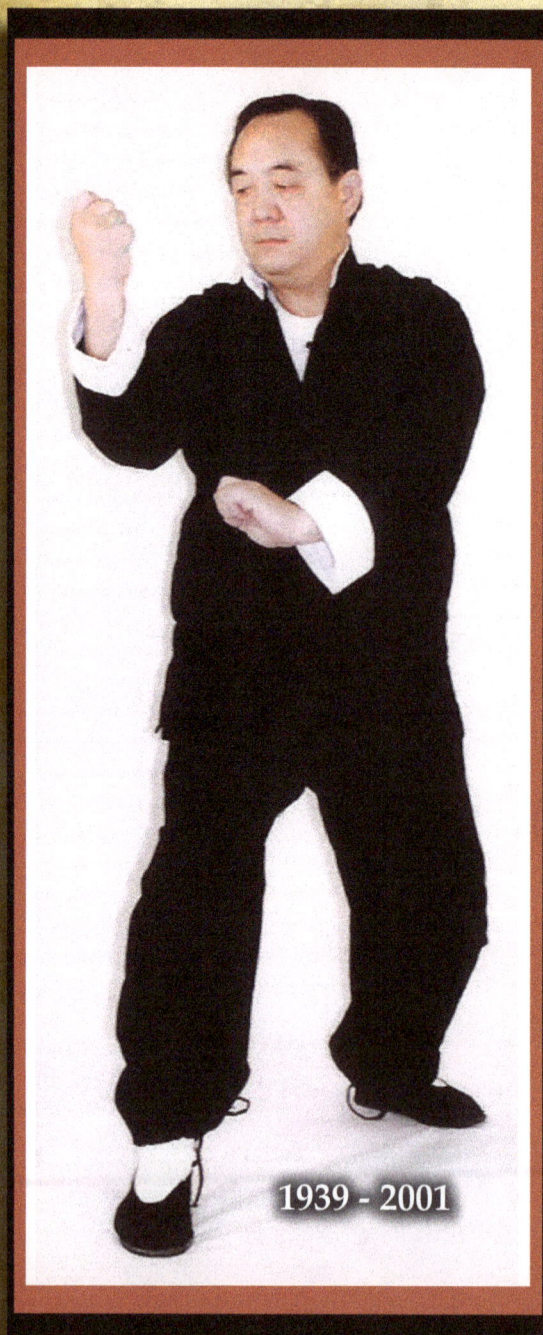

1939 - 2001

Late Sifu Gene Chen

In 1975, Master Gene Chen received certification as the first teacher of Chu Gar Praying Mantis in the United States. This certificate was awarded by popular vote of the Chu Gar Tong Long Guoshu Association of Hong Kong. Association Chairpersons were Sun Yu Hing, Dong Yat Long, and Zhang Sing.

In the early eighties, Chen Sifu stopped teaching Chu Gar boxing and began teaching Chen Style Tai Chi Chuan. He stated the style was too dangerous to teach openly. And it was also very difficult to cultivate.

Our Ancestral Shrine

Southern Praying Mantis Kungfu Creed

Hoc Yurn; Hoc Yi; Hoc Kungfu

學仁　學義　學功夫

Jurn Jow; Jurn Si; Jurn Gow Do

尊親　尊師　尊教訓　尊道義

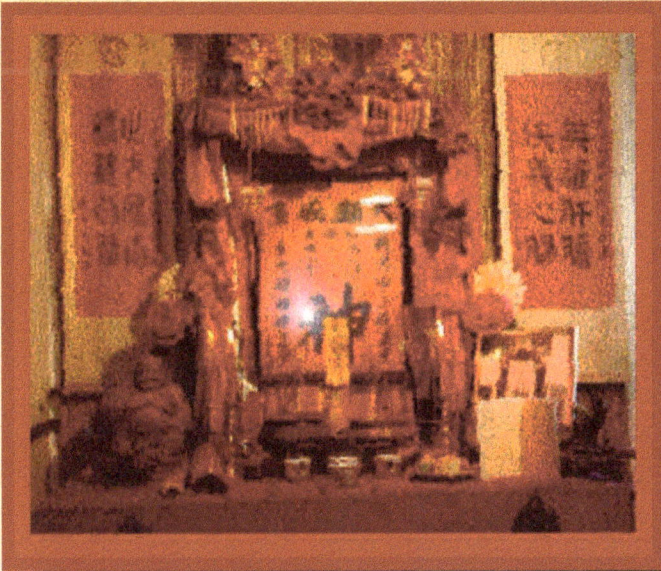

Respect the Ancestors for their transmission of the art.

Respect the Sifu for his teaching.

Respect the Older Brothers for their dedication and loyalty.

Respect the Younger Brothers for determination in training.

Contents

Front Matter

Chu Kai Ming Complete Single Man Transmission

Som Bo Gin Single Man Form - Hard Bridge

Contents

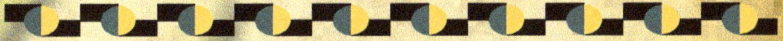

12 Basic Hand Skills

Prerequisite

Basics, in any martial art, are the beginning and end. Train the basics of Southern Mantis. Function before form. Follow step by step, at your own pace and in the convenience of your home.

Step by Step DVD Fundamental Instruction

- Volume One: Fundamentals; The Most Important
- Volume Two: Phoenix Eye Fist Attacking / Stepping
- Volume Three: Centerline Defense
- Volume Four: One, Three & Nine Step Attack / Defense
- Volume Five: Centerline Sticky Hand Training
- Volume Six: Same Hand / Opposite Hand Attacks
- Volume Seven: Sai Shu, Sik Shu, Jik (Chun) Shu
- Volume Eight: Gow Choy; Hammer Fist - Internal Strength
- Volume Nine: Footwork in Southern Praying Mantis
- Volume 10: Chi Sao, Trapping, Passoffs
- Refer to Page 105 for VOL 11 - 18 Advanced Two Man Forms

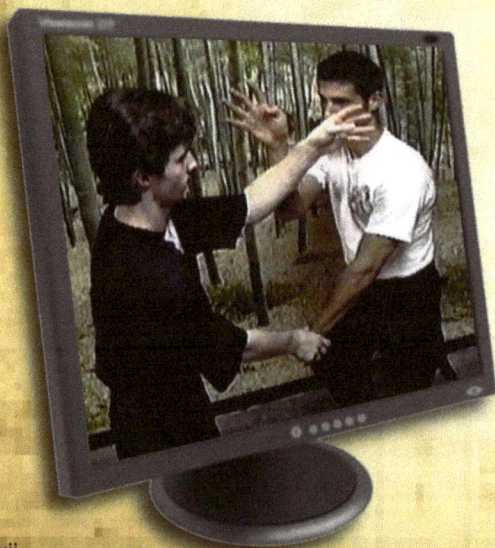

Request Volume 1 - 18 Today!

Follow Step by Step DVD Instruction

southernmantispress.com/southern-praying-mantis-instructional-dvds.htm

Book and Video

Preface

I assume you are reading this book from cover to cover and have previously read the Dedication page. Sifu Anthony Chan has many interesting stories, such as, Lam Sang (USA Kwongsai) and Lao Sui having schools opposite each other in Saukeiwan, Hong Kong. And a Northern Mantis book, in the Hong Kong Library, with a story of Lao Sui being injured by a wanderer. And the book, from 1957, that has the personal notes of Chung Yel Chong's Kwongsai Mantis and another with Chu Kwong Hua playing Chu Gar Som Bo Gin. He once had all those, but he gave them up when he went on a Buddhist pilgrimage for several years, only afterwards, to return to China Hakka Mantis, in Hong Kong.

By exchange and brother-friendship with Chan Sifu, I received the complete Chu Gar single man boxing transmission of first generation Lao Sui's disciple, Chu Kai Ming.

Special thanks to Anthony Chan Sifu, for this transmission. He shared the preliminary work, warm-ups, horse, fundamentals, basic 12 hands, and forms of this branch, with me. I am passing it on to you in this book and an upcoming DVD. But you can still join my class here, in Guangdong, China! Welcome.

It is a loss that Sifu Anthony Chan is old fashioned and prefers to remain private. However, he and I agree, the truth of Hakka Mantis is sometimes stranger than fiction, as you may read further on in this book.

In fact, instead of paraphrasing Anthony Chan Sifu's words, let me just transcribe a bit of Preface to this book, in his own words:

AC: I never had the intention of printing a book. The postures that you have used in this book are not perfect ones. I didn't do it seriously that day. If you remember, I just showed you what I have learnt from Chu Kai Ming Sifu. And you know that I have an unresolved health issue, so those postures if they are not right, just do your best to correct and explain them in the book.

RDH NOTE: We did not originally plan the film we shot to

Preface

be made into this book. The pictures herein are an accurate representation of the postures; but it was just a day of sharing and exchange with no thought to publish anything, at that time. After further consideration, however, I think it is an important work on Hakka Chu Gar Mantis that will benefit others. So, I have done my best to outline this first generation Lao Sui teaching. It is the complete Transmission of single man training, that Chu Kai Ming trained and taught from the 1920s - 1980s.

AC: By the way, I was born in 1954, and my Sifu was born in 1906. Both of us were born in the year of the horse. We were quite similar in character. He passed away in 199?. Don't know the exact year, no one knows. I heard the news from 鍾炳开 Zhong Bin Kai Sifu. He also studied under my Sifu. Another well known Hong Kong Sifu, CS Tang, was also a student of my Sifu and is my senior.

I'm quite sure you have never seen this transmission, as it has been kept private. It is a very interesting and special teaching of Chu Gar Mantis. Kwongsai and Chu are compatible. They are both Hakka Mantis and from one origin.

I was in the USA, San Jose around 1978 and I met Norman Lee, a student of Gene Chen, in San Francisco. I visited Gene a couple of times in San Francisco and he communicated with me by letters also. Norman was straightforward and honest with me.

RDH: Yes, Gene was my first Chu Gar Sifu by ceremony circa 1989. Norman and I were friendly and trained some together, but I have lost touch with him. I'm quite sure I was Gene's last Chu Gar disciple. He only ever had three or four. But, he had many Tai Chi disciples eventually.

AC: The last time I saw my Sifu was around 1984, before I moved to the Hong Kong, New Territories in 1985. Prior, I lived on Hong Kong Island and my Sifu lived there nearby Victoria Park. No one knew when he passed away because no one knew his address. Tse Chung 謝松 one of the Chu Gar Five Tigers, the first disciples of Lao Sui. Tse was my Sifu's Dui Jong training partner. It was Tse Chung who said if you know Som Bo Gin and Dui Jong, then you know

Preface

half of Chu Gar already.

RDH: I visited Cheng Wan Sifu and Yip Sui Sifu in Hong Kong, circa 1989. Cheng Wan refused to see me but I became friendly with Yip Sui for a time. In 2002, Cheng Wan accepted me by tea and appointed me a Standing Chairman of his Association with the task to carry on and blossom Chu Gar.

To that end I have been working on a comparative analysis of the various branches of Hakka Mantis: Kwongsai, Chu Gar, Iron Ox and the various clans such as, Huizhou Chu Gar, Yang's Chu Gar, Hong Kong Chu Gar and now your Sifu's transmission also. I know you have always kept from early on, very detailed notes about the teaching you received.

AC: We didn't have names for the various hands. Sifu showed us the technique and usage, but those old timers didn't say this is called so and so. Most of the names used now were either started by Tam Wah or Ip Sui because they had put them in letters. Later on people created their own names for the skills, but not all the students were educated, and the academic standard was sometimes very low.

RDH: Yes, it was the same for Lam Sang's teaching in the USA. It was his first generation of students that mostly gave the names to various hands and skills. It was like his Qigong. They applied names like "shooting a basketball" and "holding a bucket" so they could remember the postures. I will publish more on this topic in the future.

AC: Basic Hand Skills #9 and #12, (shown on the following pages), do not exist in any other Sifu's transmission, for sure. They were developed by Chu Kai Ming to fight against Karate. #9 looks like your Lop Shu Grabbing Hand, but it is blocking against round kick.

#12, those Elbows strikes, are used in fighting with Thai Boxers. In the 1970s, free fighting was very popular and many competitions between Thai and Hong Kong Kungfu were held publicly. The other skills are pure Chu Gar, for certain. Gene Chen's hand techniques were combinations of skills like ours. He had two

Preface

techniques 四門絞搥 – 四門包椿 of Four Gate form. Their stance was different.

RDH: I'm quite sure Gene Chen Sifu only had three teachers: Dong Yat Long, Sun Yu Hing, and Yip Sui. All three were second Generation of Lao Sui.

AC: All in all, we are different. The hand skills I received from my Sifu, Chu Kai Ming, are a bit different and that is why I treasure his transmission. It is based on the principles of Chu Gar passed down by Lao Sui during his early years. Lao Sui was the main proponent of Chu Gar in Hong Kong. He trained circa 1910, for 4 years with his teacher Wong Fook Go, in Huiyang, China, before coming to Hong Kong.

#1 Basic Hand technique is the theory of 偷漏 using the opponent's force. It is not only offensive. Some use only the centre and left and right are not used. But left and right gates can be used to follow and return the other's power back to them.

#2 is a technique that explains 桥来桥上过無桥自造桥 Bridging. No bridge then make a bridge. If a bridge exist, then come or go - up, down, left, right, or center according to what force they exert.

———————

RDH: Prior to this, I have published seven additional books on various clans of Hakka Southern Praying Mantis, including their origins, history and practices of fundamental, single man forms and two man training. One should endeavor to receive the original transmission of the Art as close to the source as possible. Search and prove all things.

———————

Read on now to know the complete transmission of Chu Kai Ming's single man training, then continue by studying each skill, step by step, from warmups, horse, and 12 basic hands, to form training.

Late Chu Kai Ming Sifu's
Chu Gar Mantis

Complete Transmission

of Single Man Training

CHU GAR MANTIS – CHU KAI MING

Sequential Transmission circa 1920 - 1986

Preliminary - Warmups
- Swing Arms Front and Back
- Fic Shu 1 & 2
- Wrist Curls
- Elbows Back - Open the Chest

Footwork - Horse Steps
- Advance Step - Forward and Back
- Cross Step and Up One Step
- Shift Step 45 Degrees and Up One Step
- Run the Horse (Circle Steps) 3 Forward / 3 Back

Som Bo Gin Single Man Form
- Late Sun Yu Hing Sifu's Hard Bridge Som Bo Gin
- Late Chu Kai Ming Sifu's Hard Bridge Som Bo Gin

12 Basic Hand Skills - Ji Ben Gong
1) Jiao (Gow Choy - Center, Left, Right Hammer Fist) Steps R, L
2) Lu-Dou-Ya (Jik, Mor, Bil, Gop, Duan, Narp, Jik)
3) Nian Zheng (Chuan Sao) Passoff
4) Ge (Choc Shu - Jik Shu Opposite)
5) Bao Zhuang (Palm Strike)
6) Pi-Ge-Qin Na (Pai, Gwak, Bil, Lop)
7) Yao Shou - Ying Qin (Han - Yu Sao)
8) Meng Dan Sao (Kwongsai Um Hon)
9) Gin Jian (Cum Na Gee - Lop - Jik)
10) Chum Zheng - Sai Shou (Jik-Chum, Sai Sao)
11) Yi Kup Bao Zhang (Jao Chui, Dai Shou, Cha Cheung, Pai Zheng)
12) Cha Zheng-Liande Zheng (3 Elbow Strokes)

After Som Bo Gin, it took half a year or more to train these 12 hand skills. Each of the 12 hands, was trained several weeks before moving to the next, all the while, classes started with warm-ups, Fic Shu, Horse Steps, and Som Bo Gin. Read the enclosed **Interview** chapter for more details on Chu Kai Ming's teaching.

LAO SUI'S 1ST GEN' TRANSMISSION

Sequential Transmission circa 1920 - 1986

After training the 12 Hand Skills to completion one would also train, in Chu Kai Ming's transmission:

Continued Single Man Form Training
- Tan Zhuang - Soft Bridge Som Bo Gin
- Som Gin Yu Sao - Three Shaking Bridges (not taught in later days)
- 2nd Form - An advanced skill of Chu Kai Ming's Transmission

Chu Kai Ming passed before completing his last transmission, 2nd Form. However it was said by Lao Sui's first generation disciples, "If you understand "Dui Jong (two man training)" and "Som Bo Gin Single Man form" then you already know at least half of Chu Gar Praying Mantis.

The late Gene Chen, circa 1989, taught that Lao Sui originally only taught four forms:

- Som Bo Gin - Three Step Arrow
- Som Gin Yu Kiu - Three Shaking Bridge
- Som Bond Ging Tan - Three Spring Power
- Fut Sao - Buddha Hand

Wach for my upcoming book on Chu Gar paired training. The "Dui Jong" - two man training, in Chu Gar, consists of four basics:

- Chy Sao - Single Bridge Grinding Hand
- Dui Jong - Double Bridge Strengthening
- Gow Choy - Hammer Fist and Palm Conditioning
- Mang Dan Sao - Simultaneous Offense - Defense

(See my previous three books, *Chu Gar Gao, Chu Gar Mantis, Chu Gar Skills*, for more on Dui Jong and Chu Gar training.)

This comprises the transmission of Lao Sui's first generation disciple, Chu Kai Ming. <u>Follow this outline step by step in the following sections.</u> Read on now to see more of his teaching.

PRELIMINARY WORK

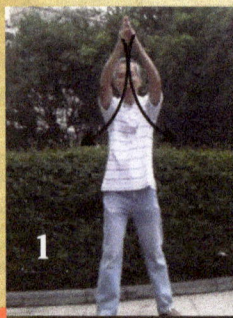

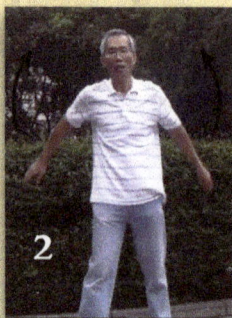

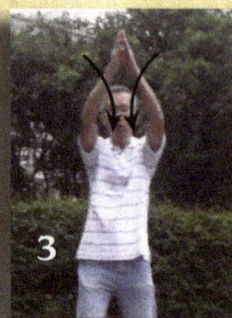

1 → FULL ARM SWINGS FORWARD AND BACK →

1-3) Swing the arms down the front and over the back18-36 times
and then repeat by reversing the direction.

After age 50, there is gradual musculoskeletal decline and injuries such as sprain,
dislocation, and tear of muscle and cartilidge are more common.

3 拂 FU—FIC SAO; FLICK, WHISK OFF BRISKLY →

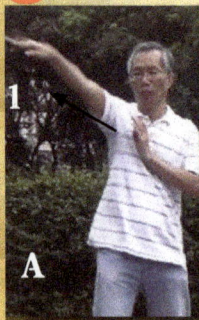

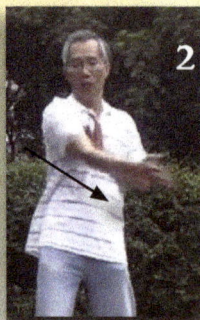

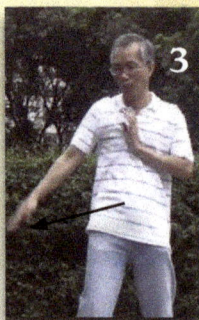

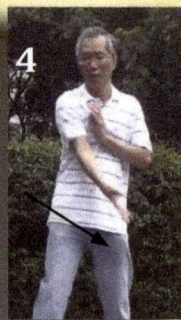

Fic Sao is found in Kwongsai and Chu Gar Mantis. The above (A) was transmitted
by Chu Kai Ming Sifu. Flick the knife-edge of the hand in the direction of the arrows.

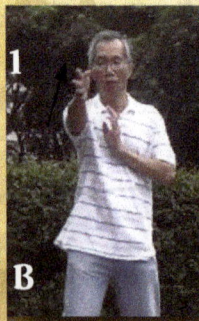

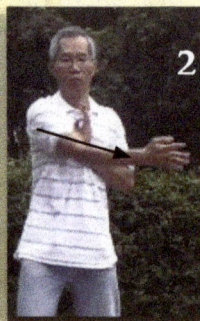

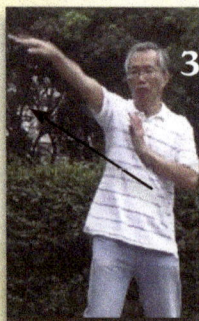

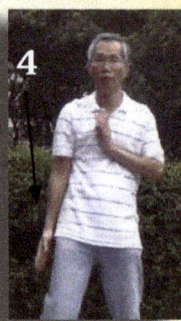

(B) was transmitted by Sun Yu Hing Sifu. Strike straight finger poke (Chop Sao)
then flick the knife-edge of the hand in the direction of the arrows.

WARMUPS 1 – 5

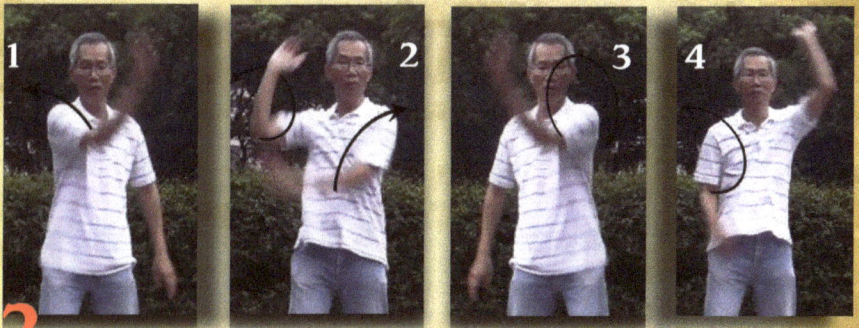

2 → **ELBOW—CIRCULAR BACK STROKES** →

1-4) Swing the crooked arms, elbows bent, in continous circles,
as if swimming the back stroke, 18-36 times.
There is less chance of injuring yourself if you are more flexible and less stiff.
Warmups become essential.

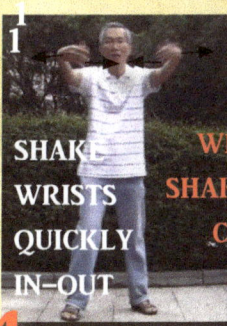

SHAKE WRISTS QUICKLY IN–OUT

WRISTS SHAKE AND CURL

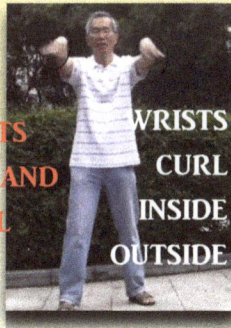

WRISTS CURL INSIDE OUTSIDE

4 →

1) Keep wrists still. Shake hands in and outward 36x.
2) Circle only wrists inside / outside 36x quickly.

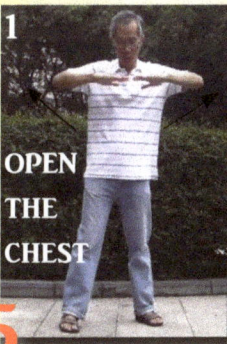

OPEN THE CHEST

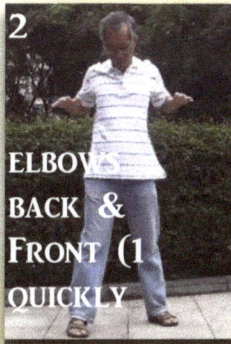

ELBOWS BACK & FRONT (1 QUICKLY

5

Push the elbows back and forward quickly 36 times.

By age 50, a person can lose 0.4 pounds of muscle every year. Sarcopenia (poverty of the flesh) cannot be escaped, but regular training can stave off injuries from muscle and bone loss. At age 80, studies show a Master Athlete has 50% loss of strength.

Perform warmups that are specific to the type of training you employ. In Hakka Mantis, shoulders, elbows, wrists, and torso are heavily employed and so the warmups shown here are useful to avoid injury.

HORSE STEPS – FOOTWORK

1 前後 FORWARD (1-3) – BACK STEPS (4)

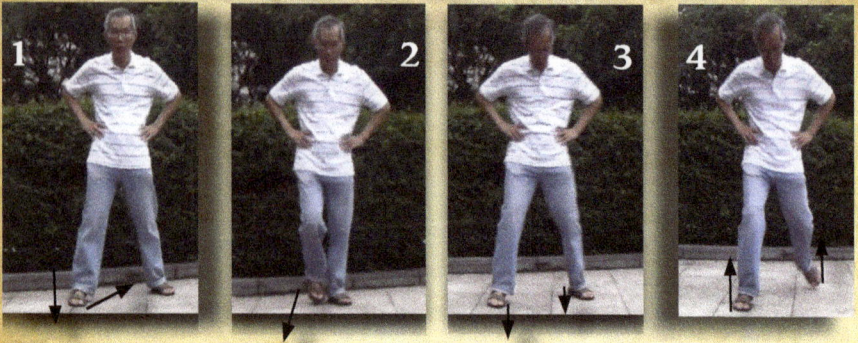

When one has understood correct Mantis posture and internal work (horse stance), he may begin to train "walking the horse" in various footwork patterns. 1-3) From right stance bring the right foot back (2) and step out and forward 6 inches straight forward (3) on the right. Repeat right forward step 36 times. Change to left step and repeat 36 times. Then alternative R-L. 4) Move the back leg rearward then front leg while maintaining stance. Repeat right, left, and alternating 36 times each.

2 CROSS STEP–STEP UP (1-5) LEFT & RIGHT

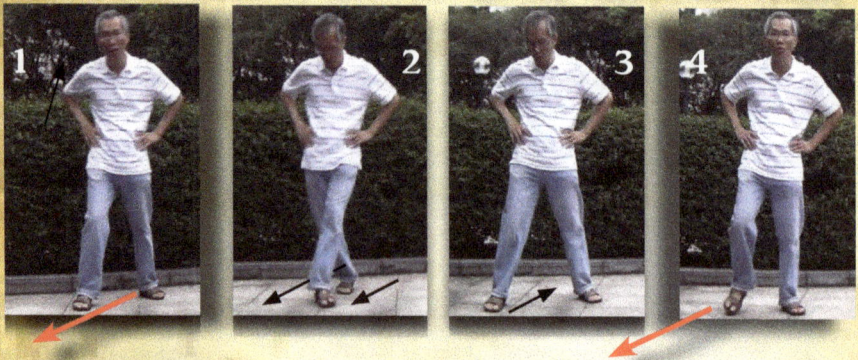

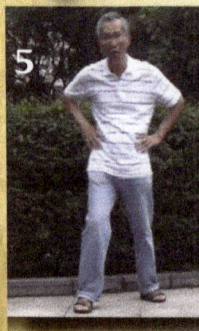

Diagonal (45°) steps are common in Mantis shadowboxing. Iron steps are firm but flexible. 1-3) Step forward at 45° crossing the back foot (2) and step upward to horse stance (3). Without pause, pull the foot back (4) and step forward 6 inches to horse stance. Repeat (1-5) 36 times right side, left side, and alternating.

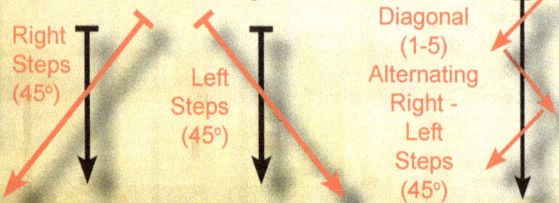

Right Steps (45°)

Left Steps (45°)

Diagonal (1-5) Alternating Right - Left Steps (45°)

HORSE STEPS – FOOTWORK

3 SHIFTING HORSE 45º OFF CENTER–STEP UP

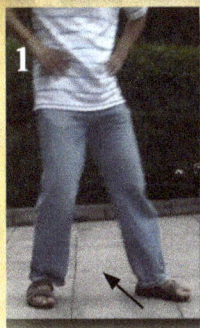

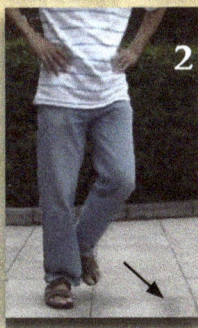

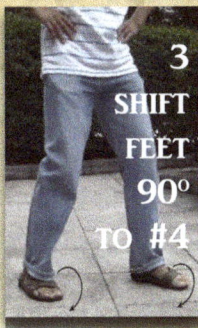

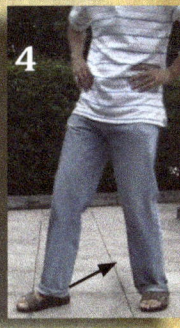

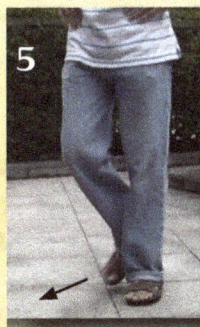

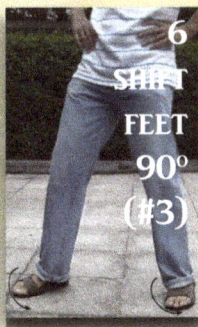

1

2

3
SHIFT
FEET
90º
TO #4

4

5

6
SHIFT
FEET
90º
(#3)

Correct horse is the father of power. Power is gathered in the legs and back and expressed in the hands. From centerline shift both feet flat footed 45º off centerline, left or right (3-4). From 45º, pull the foot back and step forward and up 6 inches on the angle - shift 90º to opposite side - repeat pull the foot back and step up on the angle - shift 90º - repeat on the opposite side - L-R - 36 times.

4 RUN THE HORSE AFTER WALKING IT

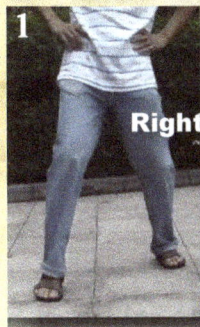

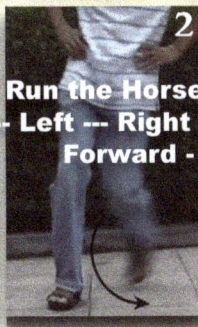

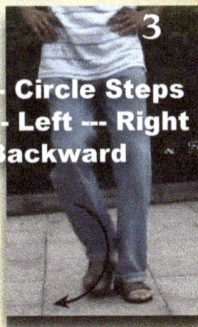

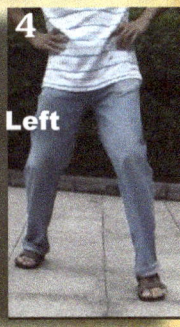

1

2

3

4

Run the Horse - Circle Steps
Right --- Left --- Right --- Left --- Right --- Left
Forward - Backward

Rooting is the skill of developing the force of a thousand pounds in the feet. With it, the stance is as firm as Mt. Tai and not easily moved. Strong legs and loose shoulders and the "chi-vital energy" will sink down to the navel. Run the rooted horse quickly three steps forward and three steps back. One may employ varied footwork patterns to run the horse. Read on now to continue with Som Bo Gin training.

Refer to the Instructional DVD: http://chinamantis.com/volume-nine.htm   23

THREE

STEPS

三步進

FORWARD

三步箭

ARROW

三步剪

SCISSORS

THREE STEPS FORWARD:
START WHERE YOU ARE.
USE WHAT YOU HAVE.
DO WHAT YOU CAN.

Your present circumstance
doesn't determine where you can go;
it merely determines where you start.

SOM BO GIN

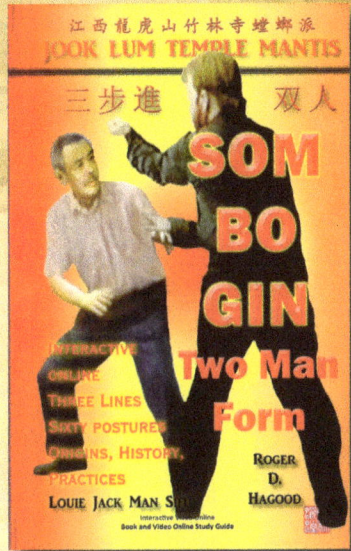

For further details about Som Bo Gin form, obtain a copy of the above book from Amazon.com or other fine online retailers.

1st Generation Lao Sui Transmission

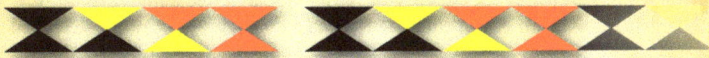

The Som Bo Gin teachings of late Sifus Chu Kai Ming and Sun Yu Hing

In the book shown above, I have offered in-depth details about Som Bo Gin, especially the two man form. I will not repeat those details herein, but, I plan a future publication which will include a comparative analysis, book and DVD, of the various Hakka factions' Som Bo Gin single man form, including Kwongsai USA and China, and the various Chu Gar factions of Hong Kong and China.

Keep in mind, there is no Som Bo Gin form, single or double man, in China's Kwongsai Mantis. Read the above book to understand this.

Different Characters - Same Pronunciation

Different traditions write the Chinese character "Gin" dissimilarly, but when pronounced they all sound the same.   As seen on the previous page, the written character "Gin" may mean "forward, arrow, or scissors", as commonly seen in Southern Mantis Kungfu.

Hard and Soft Bridge Som Bo Gin Form

Chu Gar Southern Mantis writes the Chinese character as "arrow." And the late Sifu Chu Kai Ming was innovative. He taught both a hard bridge and soft bridge version of Som Bo Gin single man form. The hard bridge was simply referred to as "Som Bo Gin". The soft bridge was referred to as "Tan Zhuang" or elastic, spring power.

To date, it is known that other first generation Lao Sui clans, such as, the Yang Clan (refer to my book *Chu Gar Skills*), also train a soft "Tan Zhuang" version of Som Bo Gin.

It seems clear that second generation Lao Sui students, which include the late Yip Sui and "his Chow Gar" did not continue this soft bridge Som Bo Gin. And today, in Lao Sui's hometown, the soft bridge form cannot be found, only hard bridge.

Author's note: I consider Lao Sui's hometown descendents, including Chen Jianming, Ma Jiuhua, and Xie Tiansheng Sifu's, hard bridge form to be the standard for Chu Gar Som Bo Gin, Three Step Arrow. See my book, *Chu Gar Mantis.*

The "Tan" in "Tan Zhuang" is common in all Southern Praying Mantis. It mean elastic force or spring power. Sometimes it is referred to as "Gan Tan Ging" or something like "frightening spring power". It is just the force that can be issued from a rooted stance through the tendons. It implies that it can stick with the opponent while following and turning his force back to him.

"Zhuang" or "Jong" as commonly seen, is the same as in "dui jong" or "muk jong" - it just means a stake or a pole stuck in the ground. So in the kungfu sense, it means the utility or function of a method - for example, in China's Kwongsai Mantis, we say the first and second fist forms are "Dan Zhuang" and "Shuang Zhuang" - it means single or double bridge training methods. Zhuang just means a method of training. "Tan Zhuang" or "Tan Jong" means the method of traning elastic spring force.

In this book, I offer you two methods of Hard Bridge Som Bo Gin, that of Lao Sui's first generation disciple, Chu Kai Ming, and that of second generation, Sun Yu Hing. Both were esteemed Chu Gar Masters during their lifetimes.

The difference is minimal between their two hard bridge versions. The Chu Gar Som Bo Gin form has three straight lines, although some would say two and a half lines. You open the form, go forward with line one, turn around, come back a second line, turn around, and come back with the third line (or 2.5 line) as a closing.

<u>The only difference between their two hard bridge versions is the third line.</u> You can see this difference in the pictorial that follows of the third line of Som Bo Gin. Sun Yu Hing's version is not only different and includes additional hands, it has a salute upon closing and Chu Kai Ming's does not have a salute. Chu Kai Ming's ends with a single bridge beggar's hand position and nothing more.

Don't take these as small nuances. These are important variations in the transmission of Chu Gar down to you today. These are esteemed masters of Chu Gar who lived from the 1920s until the 1980s. Chu Gar and Hakka Mantis was their life. It is who they were and what they did. If you endeavor to understand Hakka Southern Mantis, then understand from whence it came and what were the transmissions so that you may continue the transmission in its pure and genuine form today.

The only difference between hard bridge and "Tan Zhuang" soft bridge Som Bo Gin is that you endeavor to relax and flick out the soft elastic spring power. The form sequence is the same and the ending of Tan Zhuang soft bridge is the same as Chu Kai Ming Sifu's hard bridge (not Sun Yu Hing's third line closing sequence).

Watch for my upcoming book (and DVD) comparing the Som Bo Gin of the various clans of Hakka Southern Mantis. It will analyze in detail, step by step, the similarities and the differences of each clan and how they relate to the origins, history and practices as passed down to you since this style was created, in the mid-1800's in southeastern China!

Read on now to see the third line difference between Chu and Sun's hard bridge Som Bo Gin and view the Tan Zhuang soft bridge.

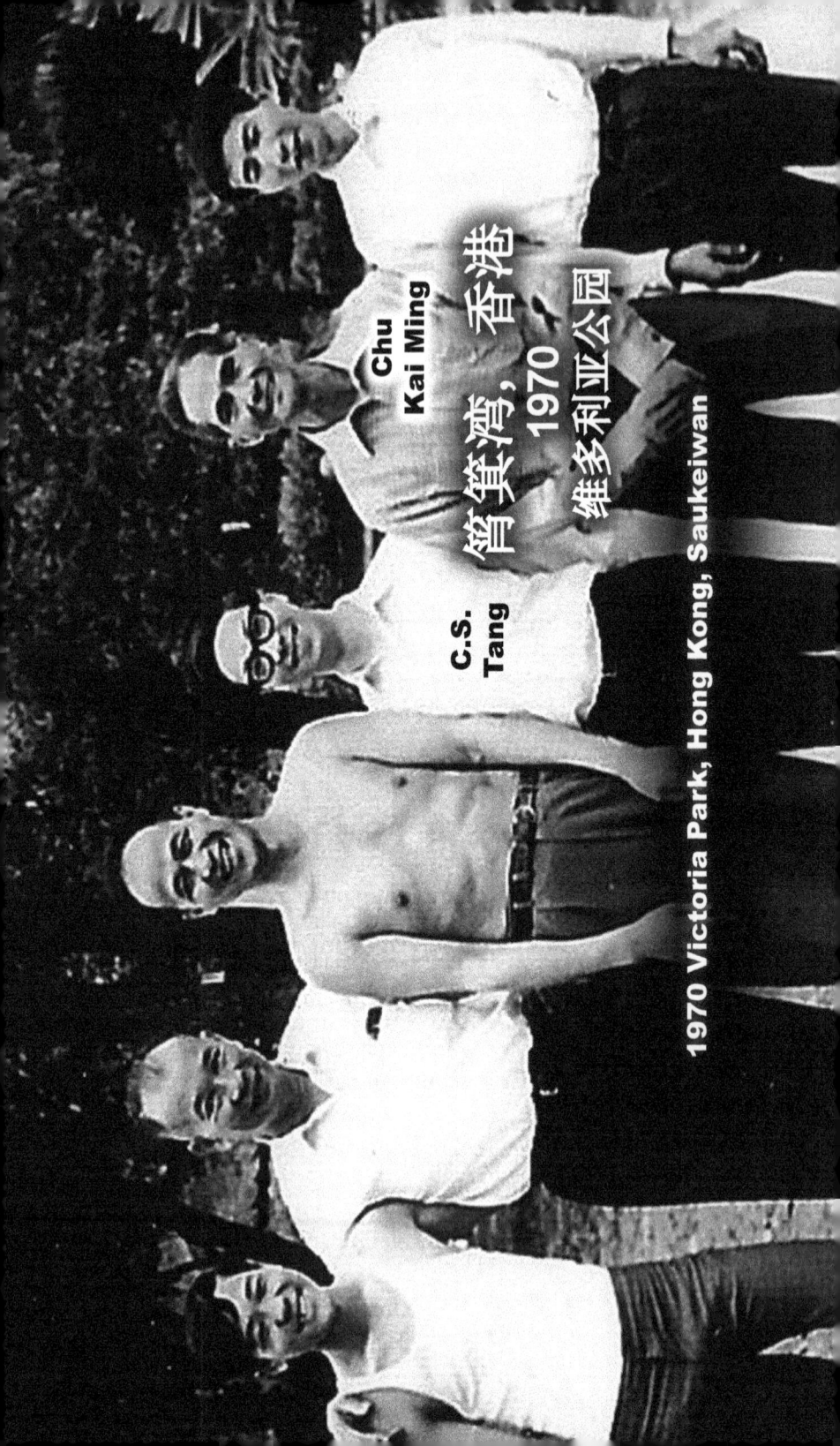

Chu Kai Ming

C.S. Tang

筲箕灣, 香港
1970
維多利亞公園

1970 Victoria Park, Hong Kong, Saukeiwan

Cheng Wan

Sun Yu Hing

Chu Kwong Hua

Cheng Chiu

1976 Chu Gar Mantis Cheng Wan Martial Art Association, Hong Kong

GAR MANTIS – SUN YU HING

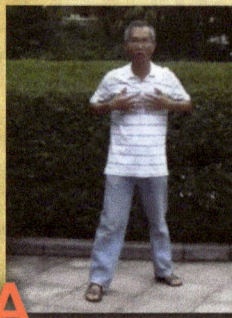

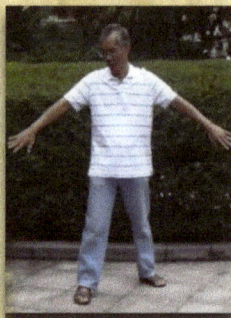

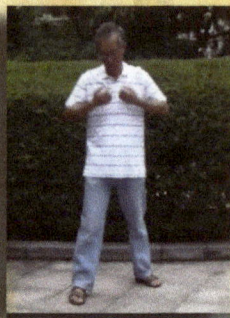

A

opening sequence - hand to hand - heart to heart

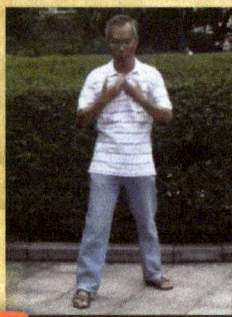

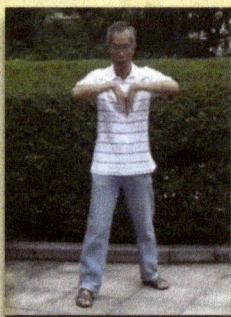

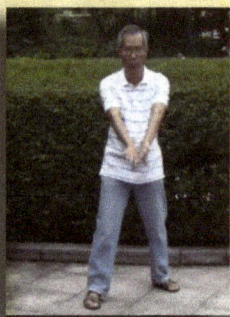

B

open and close - muscle tendon change

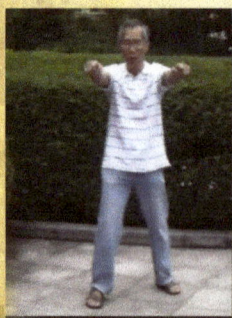

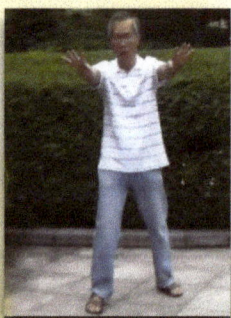

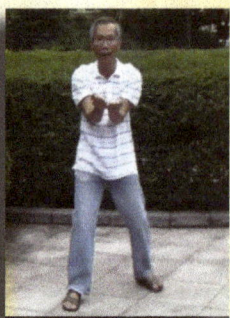

C

first three step - jik straight strikes, bil jee finger strikes, gop shu

SOM BO GIN FORM – HARD BRIDGE

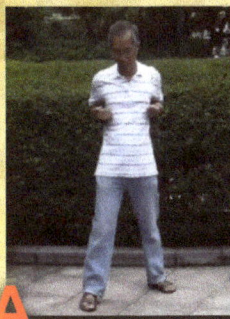

A

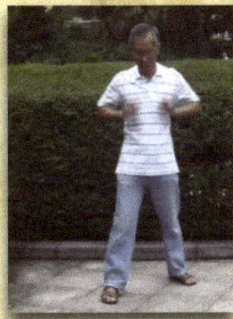

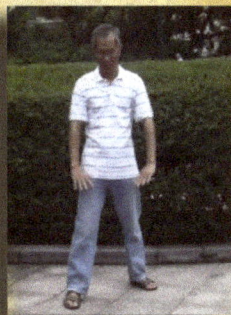

raise the stomach - compress the ribs - round the back

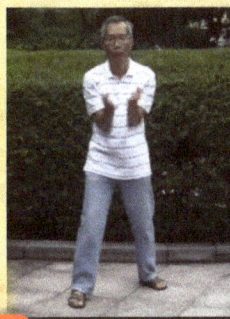

B

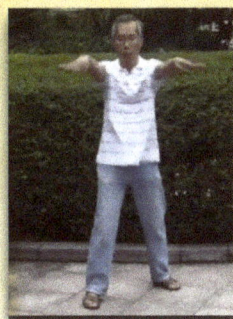

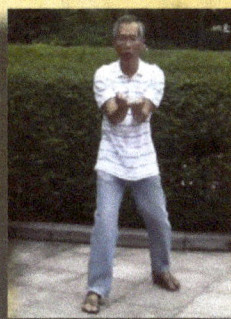

elbows inward - bil jee - gop shu

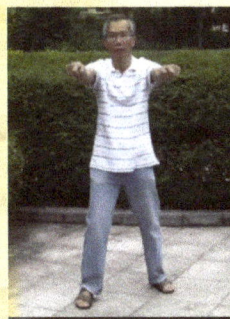

C

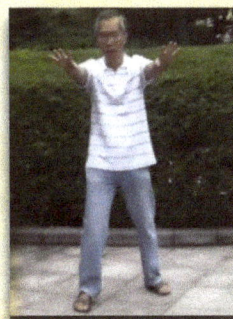

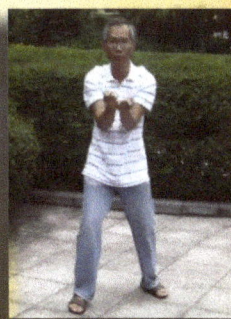

second three step - jik straight strikes, bil jee finger strikes, gop shu

31

GAR MANTIS – SUN YU HING

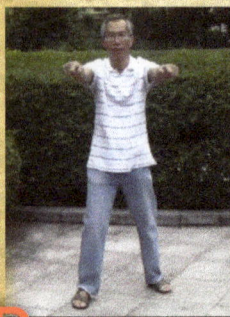

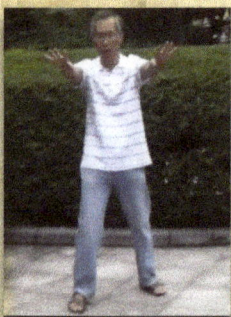

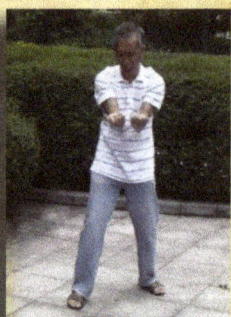

D

third three step - jik straight strikes, bil jee finger strikes, gop shu

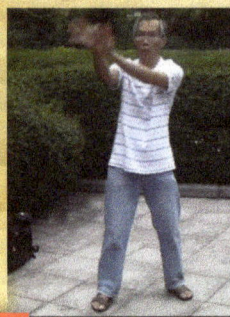

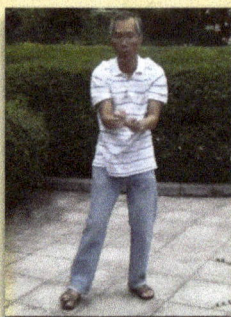

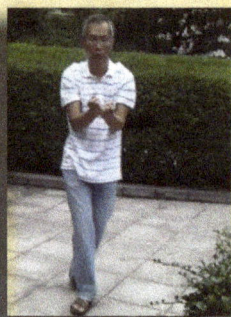

E

claw to gop shu - cross step to left

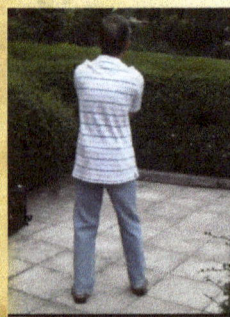

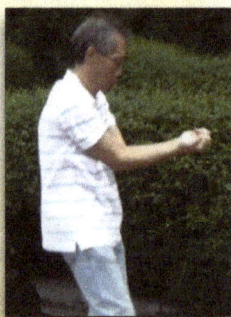

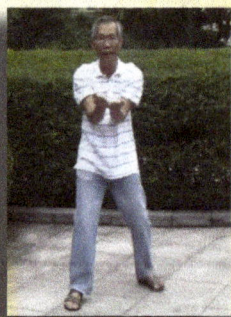

F

LINE TWO BEGINS - complete turn around with gop shu

SOM BO GIN FORM – HARD BRIDGE

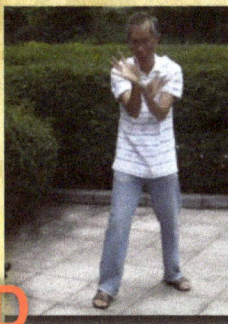

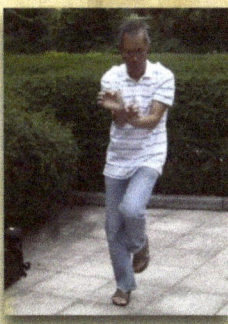

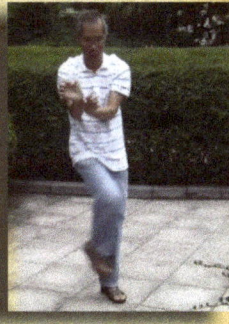

D

double claw - left, right chop steps

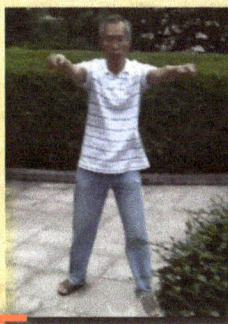

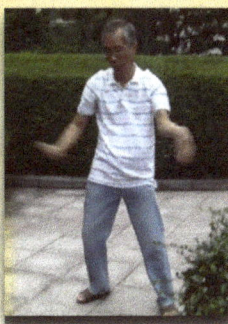

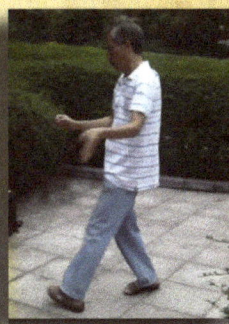

E

left foot turn around with locking hands

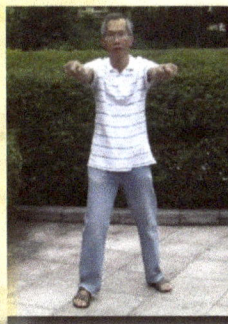

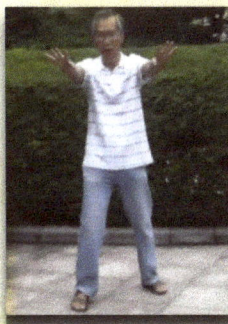

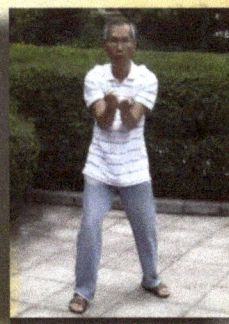

F

SECOND LINE - first three step - jik straight strikes, bil jee finger strikes, gop shu

GAR MANTIS – SUN YU HING

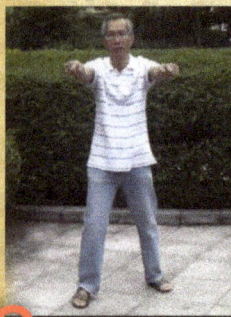

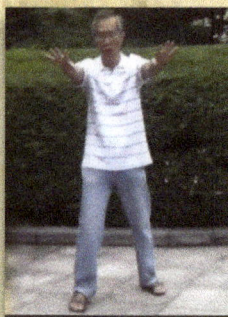

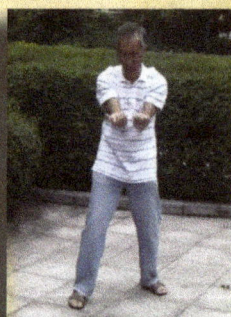

G

SECOND LINE - 2nd three step - jik straight strikes, bil jee finger strikes, gop shu

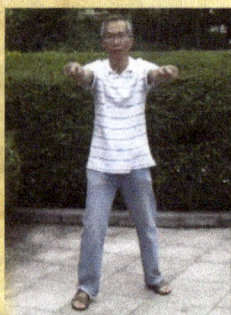

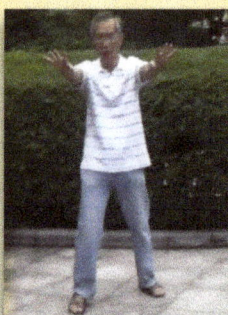

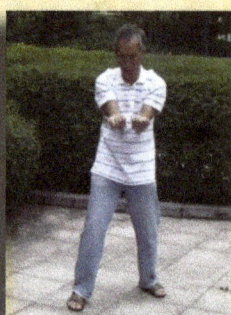

H

SECOND LINE - 4th three step - jik straight strikes, bil jee finger strikes, gop shu

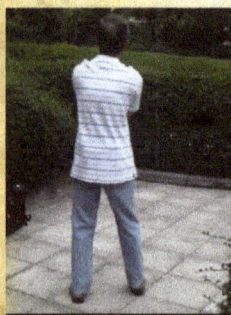

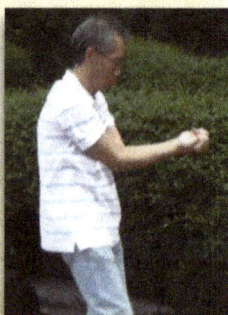

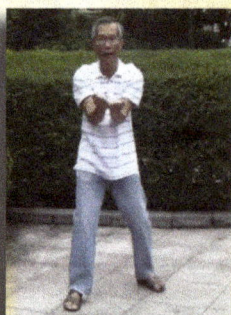

I

LINE THREE - CLOSING FORM BEGINS - complete turn around with gop shu

SOM BO GIN FORM – HARD BRIDGE

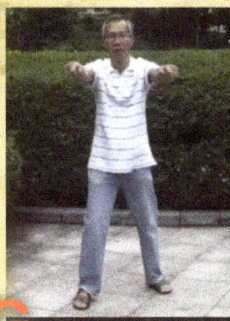

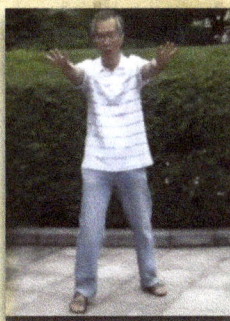

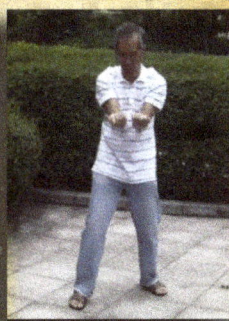

SECOND LINE - 3rd three step - jik straight strikes, bil jee finger strikes, gop shu

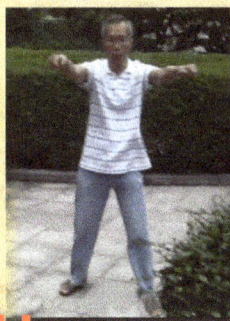

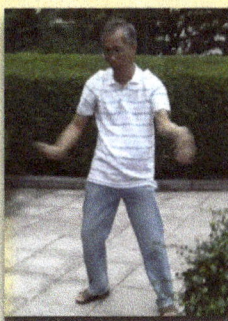

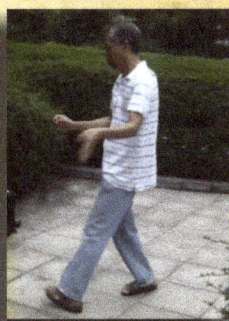

SECOND LINE - cross step - left foot up jik strikes and turn around with locking hands

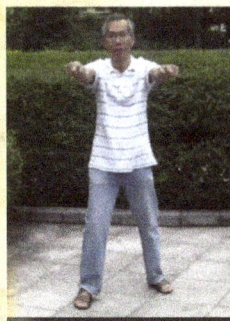

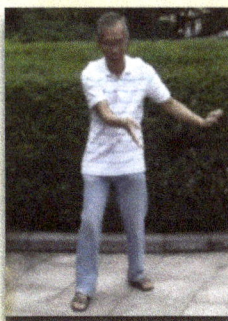

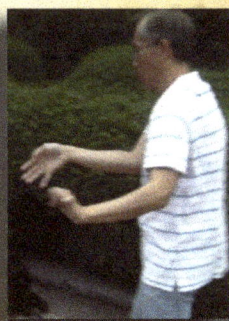

THIRD LINE - jik straight strikes, step back with locking hands

35

GAR MANTIS – SUN YU HING

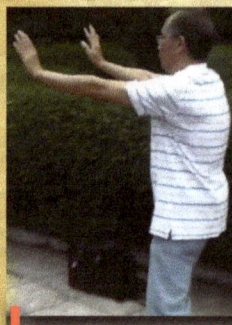

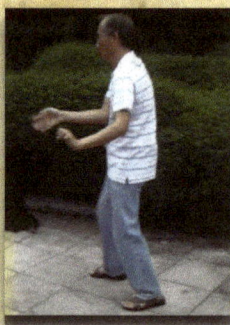

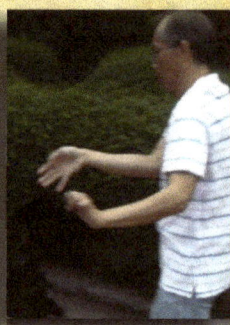

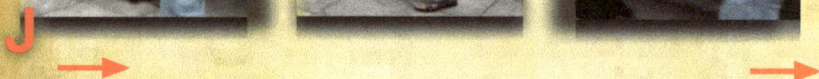

J →   →

THIRD LINE - step (R) forward double palm strikes - step back with locking hands

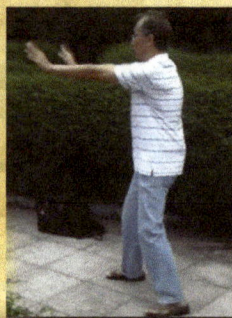

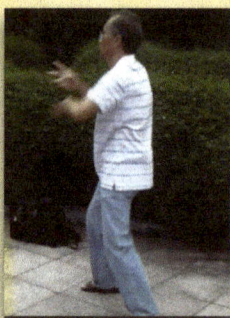

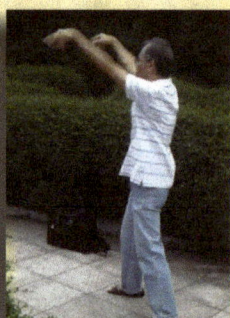

K →   →

THIRD LINE - step (R) forward double palm strikes - double pak shu up

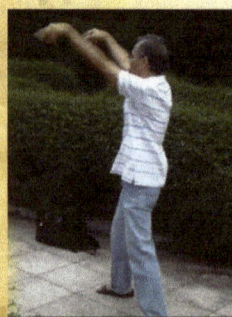

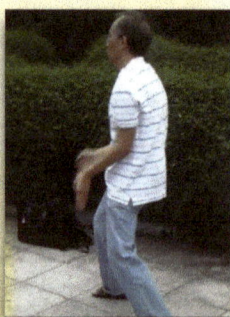

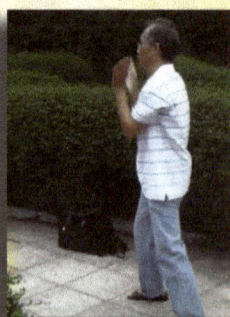

L →   →

THIRD LINE - double pak shu up, circle down to bao zhang palm (next picture)

SOM BO GIN FORM – HARD BRIDGE

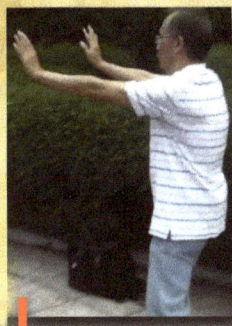

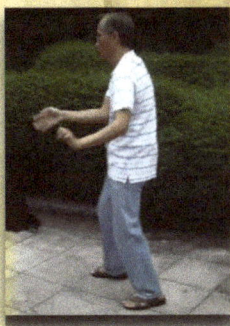

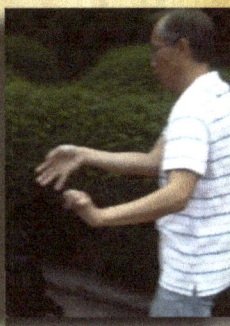

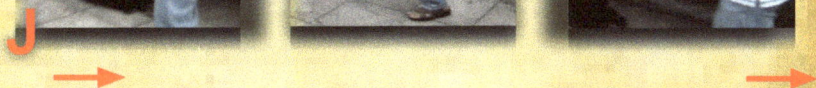

THIRD LINE - step (R) forward double palm strikes - step back with locking hand

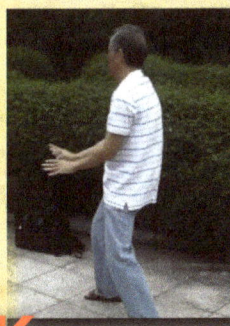

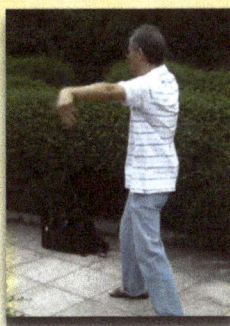

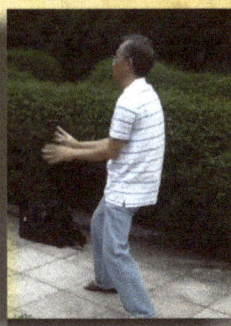

THIRD LINE - sink palms down - double pak shu out - sink palms down

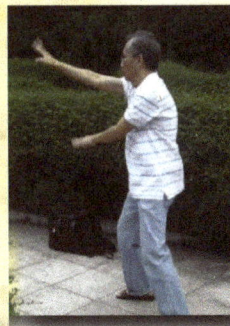

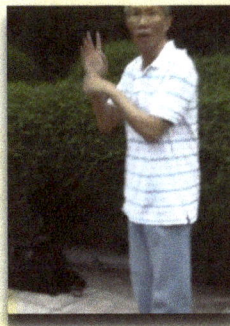

Sifu Anthony Chan teaches both a "Hard Bridge" Som Bo Gin and a "Tan Zhuang - Soft Bridge" Som Bo Gin, as shown in this book.

"Tan" translates soft or elastic power and is sometimes referred to as "frightening spring power".

THIRD LINE - bao zhang palm strike - step back feet together and salute

GAR MANTIS – CHU KAI MING

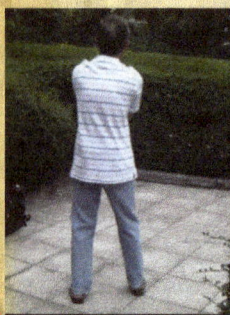

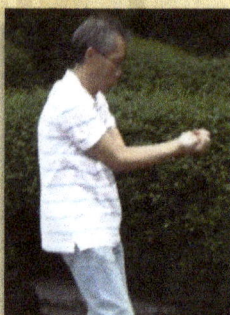

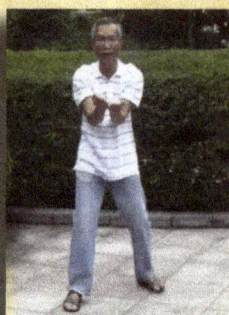

I →

FOLLOW PREVIOUS PAGES A - H:
Chu Kai Ming's Hand Bridge Som Bo Gin only differs on this line 3
Complete 2nd line turn around with Gop Shu as shown above →

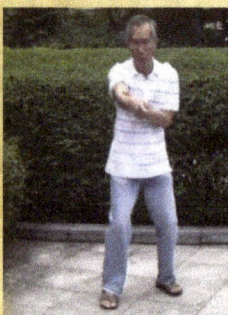

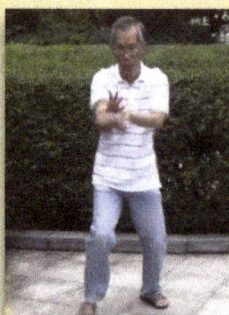

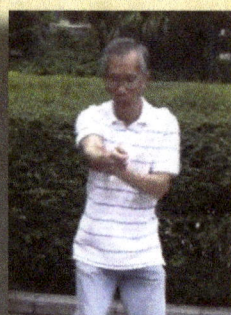

J →

THIRD LINE - step (R) forward jik shu straight strike - repeat a second time →

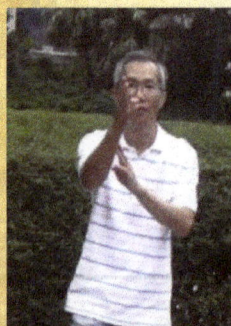

This is first generation Lao Sui transmission and this ending of the Som Bo Gin single man form can be found not only in the Chu Kai Ming teaching but, also in the first generation Yang Clan. Refer to my book, "Chu Gar Skills." I suspect this ending may be found in other first generation transmissions of Lao Sui, as well.

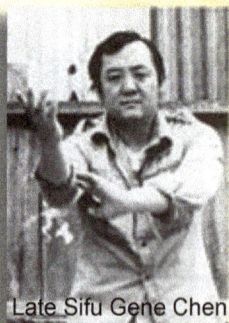

Late Sifu Gene Chen

Above: This THIRD LINE ends with single bridge Beggar's Hand Salute

SOM BO GIN FORM – HARD BRIDGE

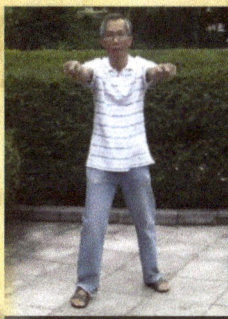

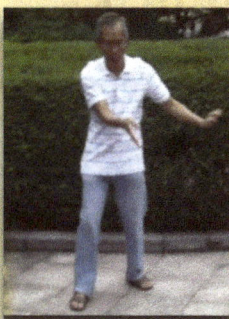

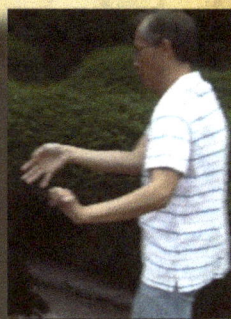

THIRD LINE BEGINS - step up - jik straight strikes, step back with locking hands,
Repeat these two actions three times on the right horse

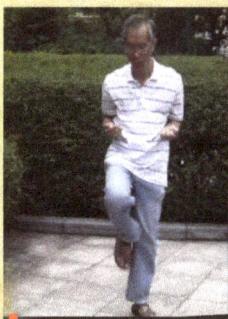

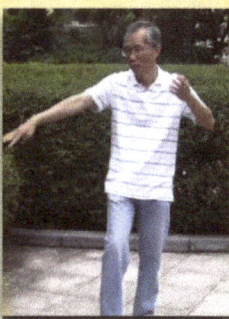

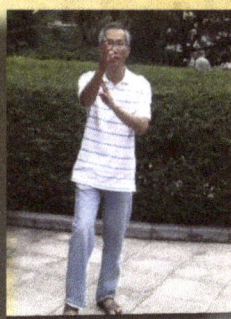

THIRD LINE - knee up elbows back - pai shu side - ending salute
(single bridge Hat Yi Sao Beggar's Hand right)

Sifu Anthony Chan teaches both a "Hard Bridge" Som Bo Gin and a "Tan Zhuang - Soft Bridge" Som Bo Gin, as shown in this book. The Som Bo Gin stepping pattern is the same for hard and soft bridge, however, soft bridge uses "Tan Li", elastic spring power, and a slightly different technique of bringing out the "arrow" power.

In hard bridge, you train to spit out the double bridge phoenix eye punch once followed by finger spears, Bil Jee. In soft bridge training, the Tan Zhuang form, you flick the hands out and forward using elastic spring force, to the same position as the hard bridge double phoenix eye punch. The primary aim in soft bridge is to relax and develop soft elastic spring power with explosive force. It is only by relaxing one may stick and borrow the opponent's hand.

SOM BO GIN – CHU KAI MING

Line One:
- Opening Sequence
- Three Step Arrow First (Right)
- Three Step Arrow Second (Right)
- Three Step Arrow Third (Right)
  (Double Bridge Phoenix Strike and Finger Pokes Bil Jee)
- Double Circle Mor Sao (Cum Na)
- Double Knees Up - Left, Right - Gop Shu
- Cross Step - Left - Double Jik Shu - Locking Hands
- Turn Around - Gop Shu

Line Two:
- Three Step Arrow First (Right)
- Three Step Arrow Second (Right)
- Three Step Arrow Third (Right)
- Three Step Arrow Four (Right)
- Cross Step - Left Step - Double Jik Shu - Locking Hands
- Turn Around - Gop Shu

Line Three:
- Step up Right - jik straight strikes, step back with locking hands;
  Repeat these two actions three times on the right horse
- Step (R) forward jik shu circular straight strike -
  repeat a second time
- Knee up elbows back - pai shu right side - ending salute -
  (single bridge Hat Yi Sao Beggar's Hand right)

SOM BO GIN – SUN YU HING

SOM BO GIN ONLY LINE THREE CHANGES:
- LINE THREE - - complete 2nd Line turn around with gop shu
- jik straight strikes, step back with locking hands
- step (R) forward double palm strikes - step back with locking hands
- step (R) forward double palm strikes - step back with locking hand
- step (R) forward double palm strikes - double pak shu up
- sink palms down - double pak shu out - sink palms down
- double pak shu up, circle down to bao zhang palm
- bao zhang palm strike - step back feet together and salute - form ends

Note: Sun's locking hands move in a sweeping arc instead of directly.

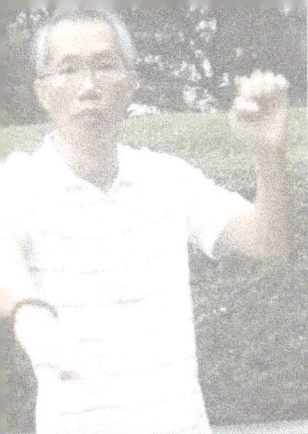
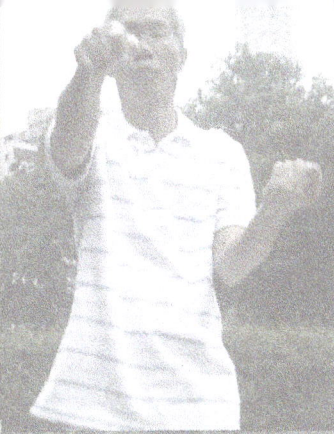
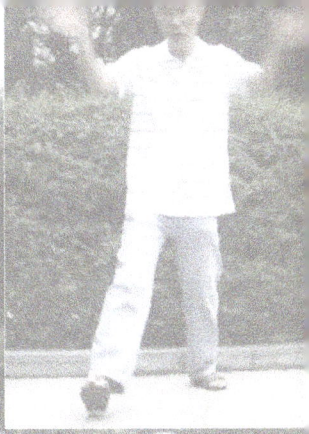
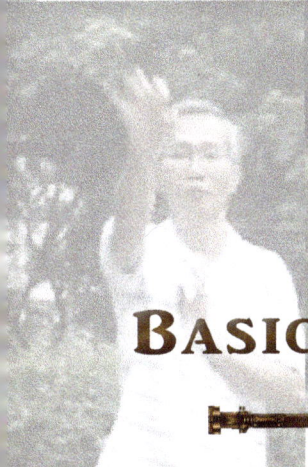
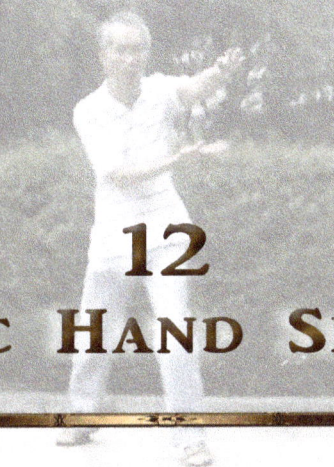
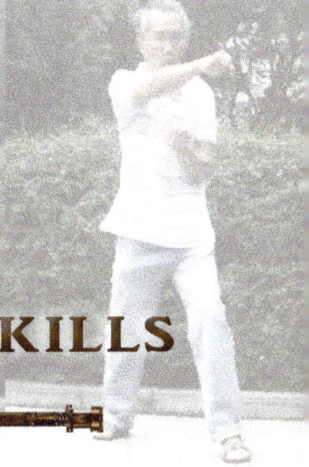

12
BASIC HAND SKILLS

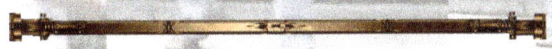

基本功

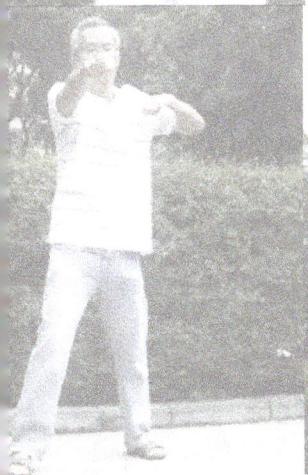
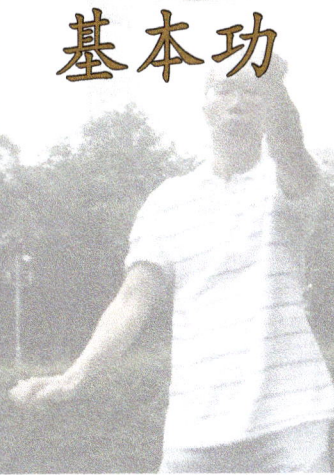
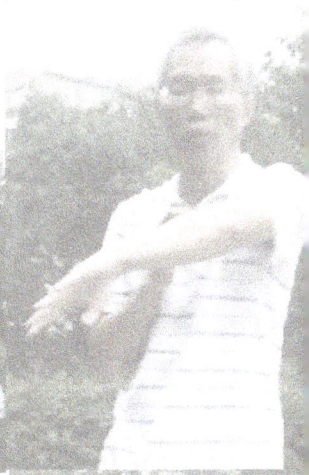
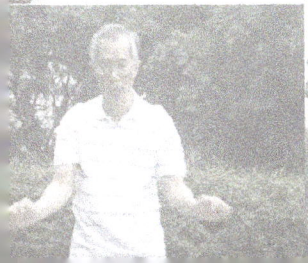
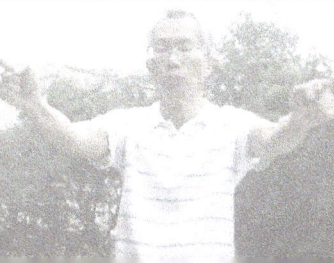
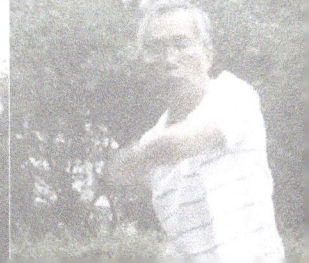

INTRODUCTION OF 12 BASIC SKILLS

Summary of Mantis External Work

- 擒拿 **Qin Na** - grasping, seizing of joints, bones, muscles, tendons, circulation
- 揸捉 **Jia Jook** - clutching, holding with the fingertips
- 批割削 **Pi Ge Qiao** - offensive, defensive bridge hands

Summary of Mantis Internal Work

- 吞吐浮沉 **Tun, To, Fo, Chum** - swallow, spit, float, and sink power
- 驚彈勁 **Gan Tan Ging** - frightening spring power, elastic power

Introduction by Anthony Chan Sifu

散手 San Sao is a term used in the old days. It refered to any fighting techniques, single or in a series, like 12 hands (手) in Chu Gar, or 18 basic hands (手)(Buddha Hands) in Kwongsai Mantis. A lot of people trained 散手 San Sao to protect themselves. I knew one guy who learned from Sun Hing and spent ten years in order to train the San Sao 散手, even though he only learned a few hands. 散手 San Sao, the basic fighting hands, were always taught privately. Only forms were used to perform in the public. It is kind of sad, because this kind of teaching will soon be lost in the world.

My Sifu, Chu Kai Ming's 12 basic hands are rather unique and differ from most other clans in that these fundamental skills are not static single hand actions - each of the 12 basic hands has several different actions combined into one hand.

When I began training with Chu Sifu, we started every day with warm ups, then 行馬 horse steps, 三步箭 Sombogin, 对双椿 Dui Jong Crossing Hands, 搓手 Grinding Hands, and 搓馬 Grinding Horse, for about an hour. Only then, Sifu would show you the 散手 San Sao basic hand skills. If you knew all of them, you would assist him in teaching. We only practiced all 12 hands in private or in front of Sifu for correction, not in public.

Sifu then will 摩手 Mor Sao feeling hands with you, a kind of sparring. He called this 喂手 Wei Sao - feeding you with the techniques. It seems gone with time. Nowdays it seems totally different—seems people like forms and dances more.

BASIC FIST FORMS

Tiger's Mouth
Ma Jiu Hua Sifu
Huizhou Chu Gar

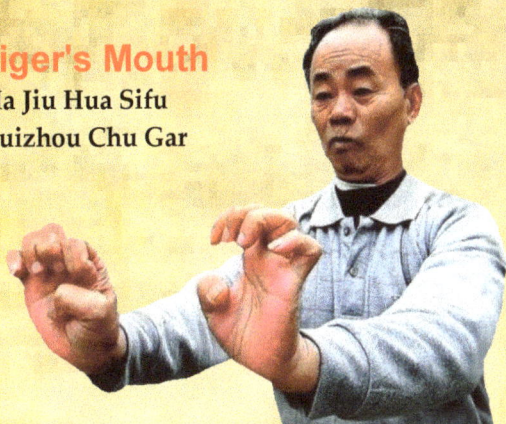

Tiger's Mouth is the grip space between the thumb and the index finger. One should be able to crush a walnut in the Tiger's Mouth. In Chu Gar the fist is closed finger by finger beginning with the Tiger's Mouth, middle finger, ring finger, and last the little finger.

Phoenix Eye
Chen Jian Ming Sifu
Huizhou Chu Gar

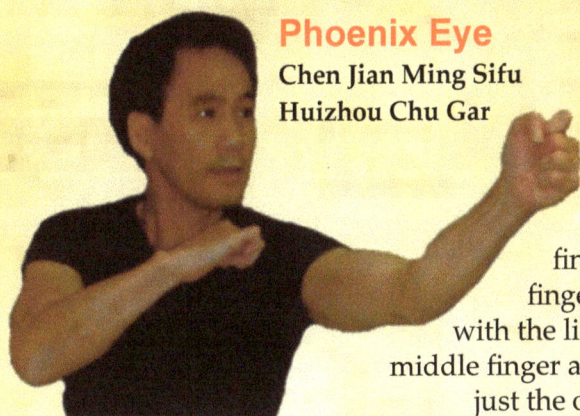

Phoenix Eye Fist is the protruding middle kunckle of the index finger. It is supported by a tightly closed thumb against the middle finger. The fist is closed finger by finger beginning with the little finger, ring finger, middle finger and phoenix fist form - just the opposite of closing the Tiger's Mouth.

Ginger Fist

Fists formed in the shape of a ginger root.

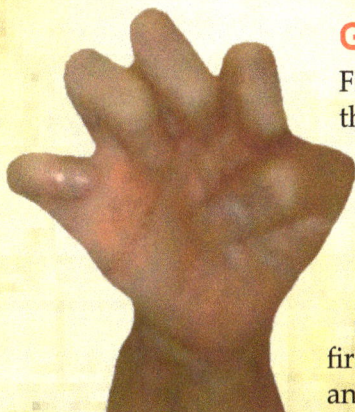

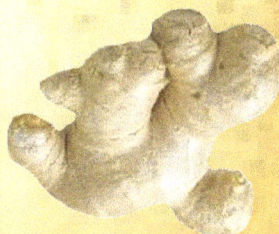

ginger root

Function is striking and slicing with first and second knuckles, scraping, and clasping with finger tips.

43

12 Basic Hand Skills – #1

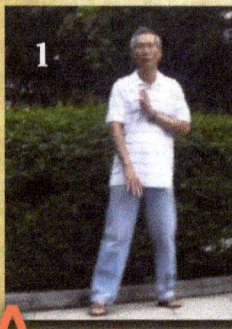

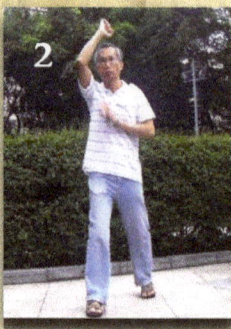

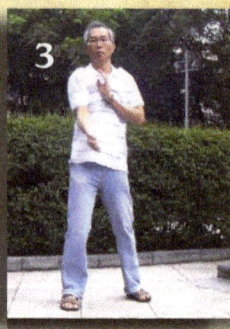

A → ← →

Right Step - Right Fist: 1) Buddha Palm Posture, 2) Big Hammer Fist over, 3) split down the middle or centerline

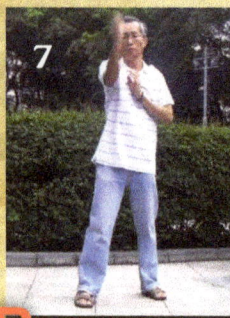

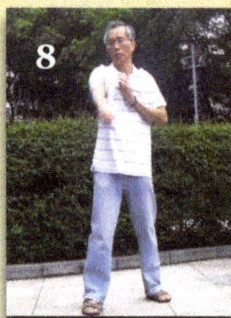

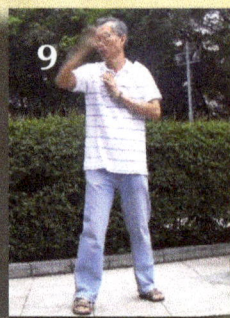

B → → →

7) Pivoting in a circle from the elbow only, 8) hammer strike downward the facing opponent's left side of the face, 9) pivot from the elbow exactly 90° right

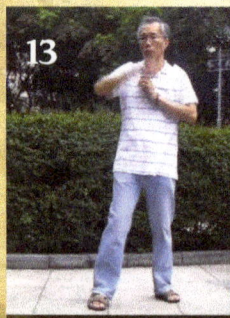

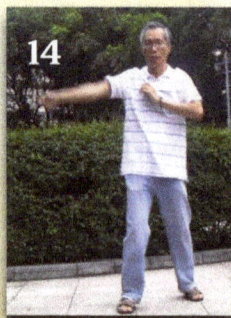

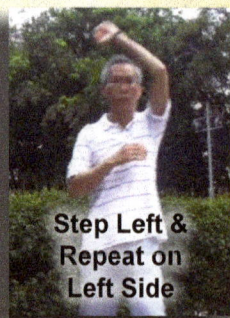

Step Left & Repeat on Left Side

C → → →

After 14) then step forward left and repeat the entire sequence on the left side, then continue alternating the steps-sequence right and left 36 times

绞 GOW CHOY—HAMMER FIST

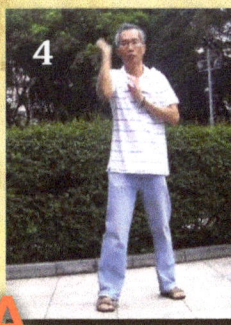

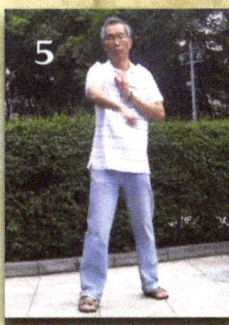

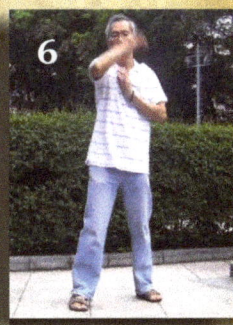

A

4) Pull elbow rearward slightly and 5) hammer strike downward the facing opponent's right side of face, 6) pivot only from the elbow and execute 7-8

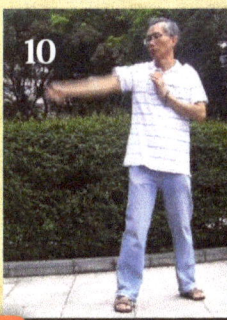

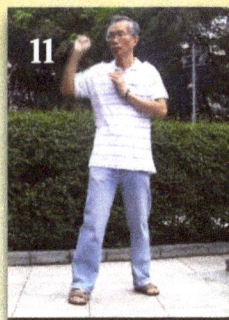

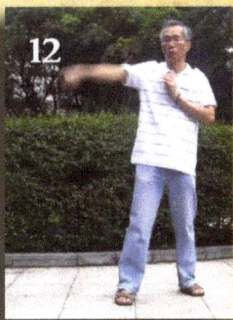

B

Repeat the big hammer fist downward strike splitting the 10) middle, 12) right side of facing opponent's face, 14) left side of opponent's face

GOW CHOY - CONTINUOUS HAMMER FIST

Gow Choy Hammer Fist is one of the main tools of Southern Mantis. There may be Big Hammer strikes (full swing) and Little Hammer strikes (which pivot and swing only from the elbow or wrist turns). The above sequence of continuous hammer strikes starts on the right foot and hand and splits the middle or centerline, right side of the facing opponent's head, left side of the opponent's head, repeats the same 90 degrees at the right shoulder before stepping forward on the left and striking the entire sequence with the left hammer fist. Each right or left step has six hammer fist strikes: centerline, right of centerline, left of centerline, 90° to the shoulder centerline, right, left (then repeat on the opposite foot and hand).

12 BASIC SKILLS – #2 将抖押

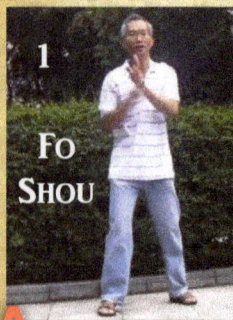

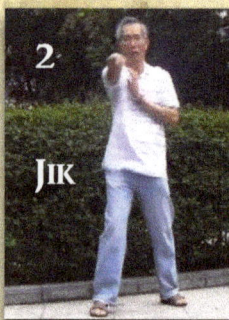

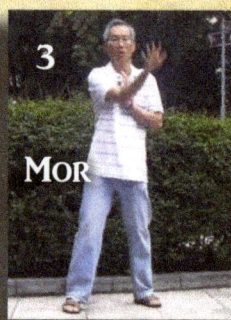

Right Step - Right Fist: 1) Buddha Palm Posture, 2) Phoenix Fist Straight Strike,
3) from fist strike circle inside Mor Sao

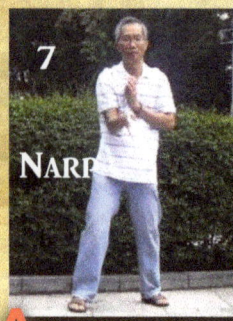

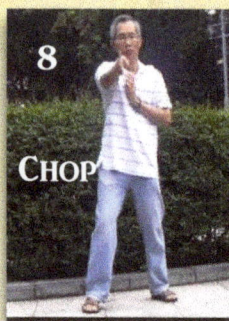

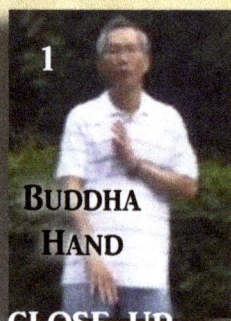

7) Sink the elbow to single bridge Narp Sao locking hand 8) immediate Chop Shu
Finger Poke. These 8 continuous actions are the 2nd Basic Hand Skill.

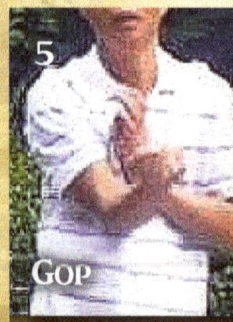

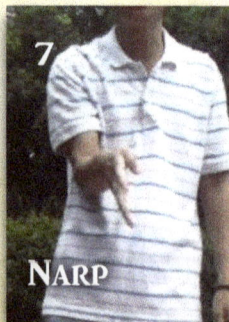

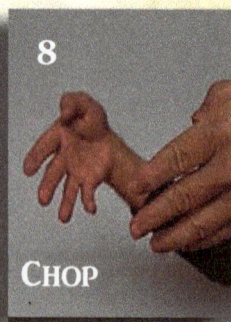

Inset photographs illustrate hands in detail. Refer to my book, "Eighteen Buddha
Hands" for an in-depth understanding of basic hand skills. Refer to Narp Sao previously.

JIK, MOR, BIL, GOP, JIK, NARP, CHOP

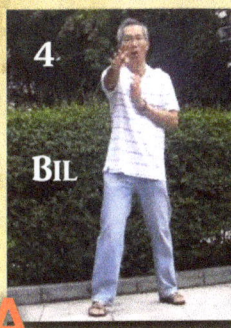

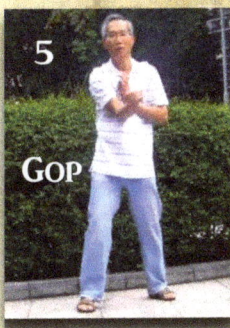

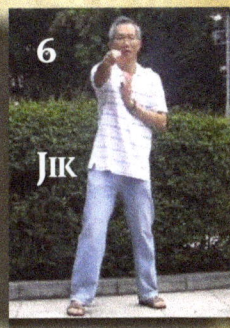

A

4) from Mor Sao immediate Bil Jee finger spear 5) change to single bridge Gop Shu Capturing Hand 6) immediate Phoenix Eye Straight Strike

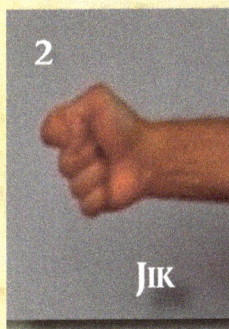

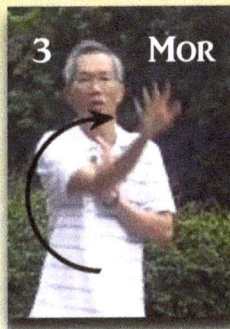

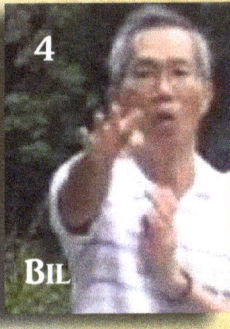

Right step-right hand-8 Actions. Then step left-left hand-8 actions on left side. Repeat 36 times alternating left and right.

BASIC HAND SKILL #2

All of the basic hand skills start with the Buddha Hand posture. This may be single or double open hands placed in front of the chest or one in chamber or resting over the abdomen. You then step right and execute seven right hand actions. Next step left and repeat the seven hand skills on the left side. Continue by alternating right and left for 36 steps. I am using the common names of each hand which follows my previous eight Southern Mantis books. However, the Chinese characters refer to the actual names which Chu Kai Ming transmitted to Chan Sifu. Refer to my "Eighteen Buddha Hands" book for in-depth details on the individual hand skills. Watch for the instructional DVD that will accompany this book teaching each of the skills shown herein.

12 Basic Skills – #3 拈挣 传手 背剑

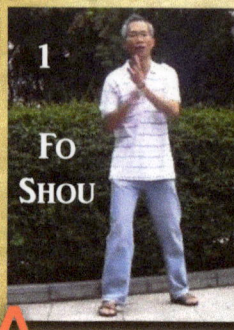

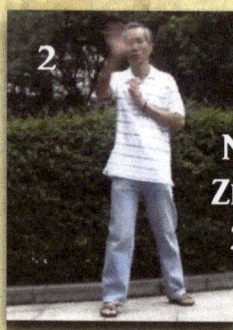

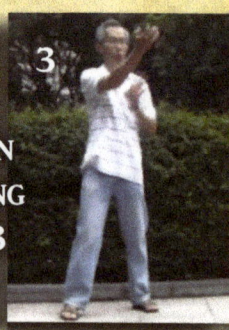

See the close-up images below. Right Step 1) Buddha Palm Posture, 2-3) **Nian Zheng** - 2) circle (wax off) right and catch with Mantis Claw the opponent's left wrist, 3) twist the opponent's left arm up and left

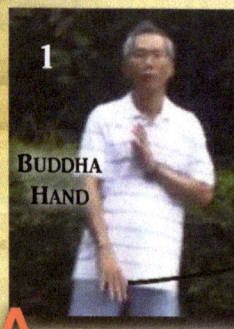

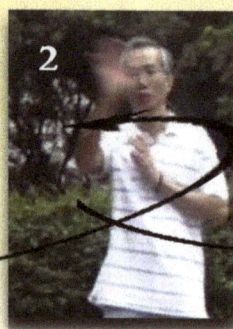

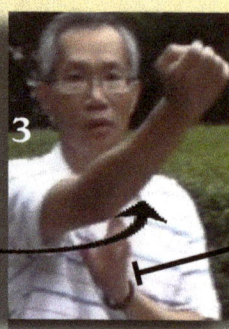

Alternate Right Step-Hand & Left Step-hand 36 times

BASIC HAND SKILL #3

Skill 3 is composed of Nian Zheng and Chuan Sao. These hand skills are common to all Chu Gar Mantis clans, but are not found in Kwongsai Mantis.   Chuan Sao is a 'passoff' - you transfer control of the opponent's arm from your right hand to your left or vice-versa. It is using two hands to control the opponent's single arm.

Kwongsai Mantis has several 'passoff' skills. However, they differ from Nian Zheng-Chuan Sao.   The Nian Zheng is a circular twist of

NIAN ZHENG, CHUAN SAO, PASSOFF

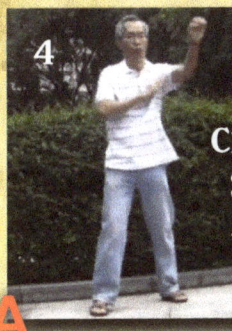
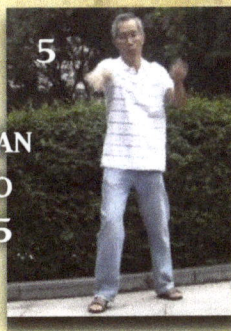

CHUAN
SAO
4-5

A ➡

4) **Chuan Sao** - passoff under your right hand while catching and lifting the opponen's wrist with your left hand 5) Hold the opponents left arm up and strike "Pai Sao" knife-edge hand to the opponent's ribs.

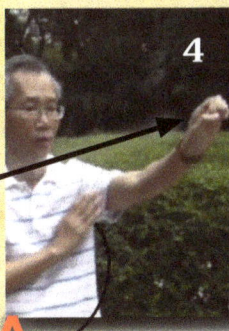
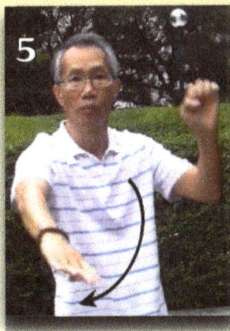

A ➡

ABOVE SHOWS RIGHT SIDE ONLY 1-5

SKILL #3 Cont'd

the opponent's wrist - arm while lifting up and across. Chuan Sao then is a passoff to your opposite hand continuing to hold or lift the opponent up and across. This is done with a simultaneous knife-hand strike to the rib cage (bottom of the 11th rib).

This method is better shown in an upcoming DVD.

Visualize 2) Catch the opponent's left wrist with your right claw - 3) twist his arm, in a circle, up and across to your left -4) passoff to your left claw lifting up and holding the opponent in place while simultaneously striking the opponent's rib cage with the right knife-hand. This right step and actions 1-5 complete hand skill #3. Now step left and starting with the left hand, repeat actions 1-5 on the opposite side. Afterwards, continue training by alternating right - left thirty-six times.

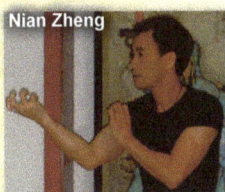

Nian Zheng

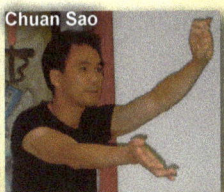

Chuan Sao

Left) Chen Jianming Sifu of the Las Sui Huizhou City Clan of Chu Gar Mantis demonstrates the twisting Nian Zheng and lifting, crossing, striking Chuan Sao actions.

12 BASIC SKILLS – #4 格

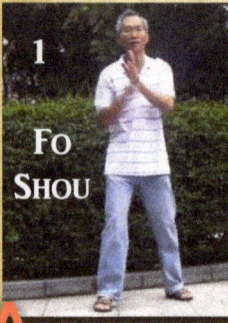

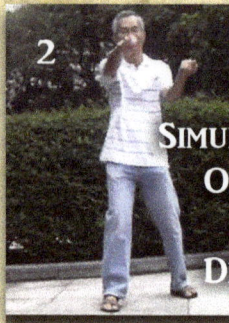

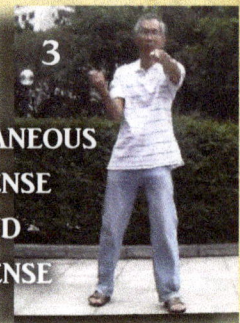

See the close-up images below - simultaneous Choc Sao - Jik Sao 1) Buddha Palm Posture, 2) step right - left Choc Sao simultaneous right jik sao phoenix eye straight strike 3) step left - right Choc Sao simultaneous left Jik Sao phoenix eye straight strike - (bottom right diagram) Choc Sao upper hooking actions control the centerline middle gate to upper gate hooking from the center outward.

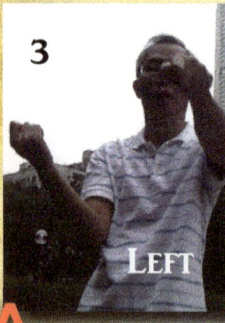

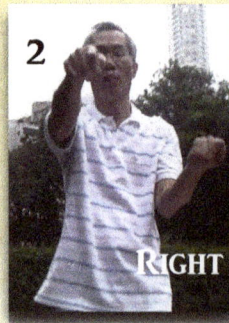

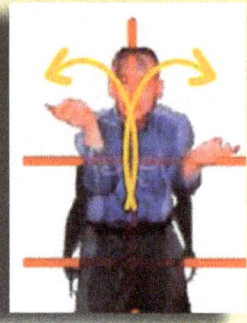

ALTERNATE RIGHT SIDE – LEFT SIDE 36 TIMES

BASIC HAND SKILL #4

Hand skill 4 is also found in the USA Kwongsai Mantis 2 man set of Loose Hands 2 and also in the China Kwongsai Mantis single man set of Say Mun Four Gate and Ba Mun Eight Gate.

#4 is a Choc Sao defense and simultaneous opposite hand attack with Jik Sao Straight Phoenix Eye Strike. You should repeat this basic exercise 36 times alternating steps right, left, right, continuously.

Remember many of the Mantis hands may be defense only, defense

CHOC SAO – JIK SAO OPPOSITE

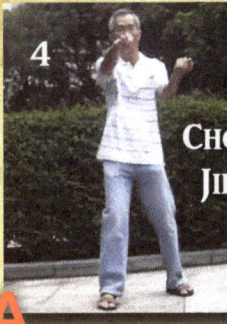

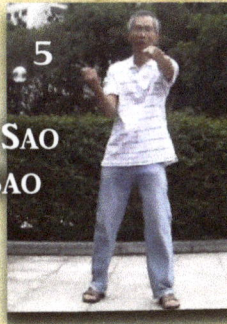

CHOC SAO
JIK SAO

A

4) step right - left Choc Sao simultaneous right Jik Sao phoenix eye straight strike 5) step left - right Choc Sao simultaneous left Jik Sao phoenix eye straight strike - repeat this continuously alternating R-L 36 times.

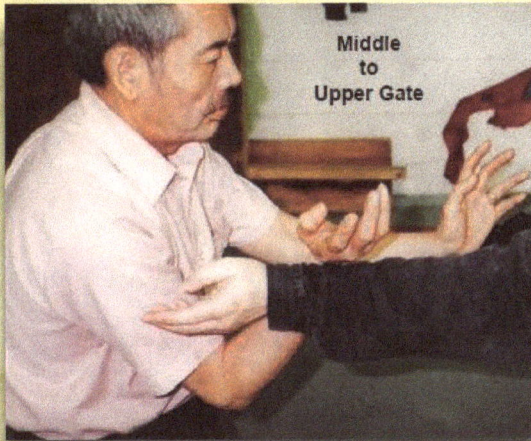

Middle to Upper Gate

Late Sifu Louie Jack Man demonstrates open hand "Choc Sao" and simultaneous "Bao Zhang" plam strike

SKILL #4 Cont'd

and counter-strike with the same hand, defense and simultaneous counter-strike with the opposite hand, as in this #4 method.

This "Choc" defense may be open hand "sao" or closed fist "choy". Open hand is "Choc Sao" - closed fist is "Choc Choy". Shown 2-5 is Choc Choy fist.

The maxim, "the arm is no match for the thigh—the weaker cannot contend with the stronger does not apply to Hakka Mantis which uses slight angles and deflections, borrowing force rather than meeting force against force.

- Choc Sao opens the centerline outward. Hook with the inner wrist across the centerline up and out from the solar plexus to the upper gate (head).
- Attributes: Slicing not banging. Hook from the forearm and slice back to the wrist.
- Function: Centerline defense, Inside, Outside, Upper and middle gate, Single bridge, Double bridge.

12 BASIC SKILLS – #5 包桩

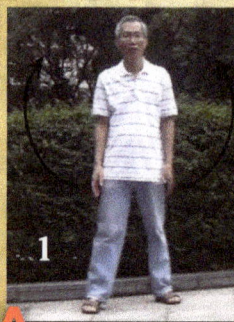 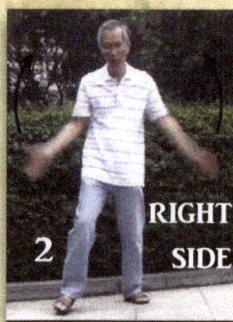 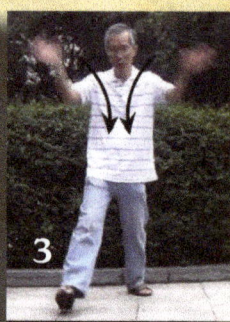

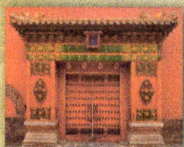

See the close-up images. The hands are a pair of Chinese doors (double doors). Open the doors–invite them in; Close the doors–throw them out, is a Hakka boxing maxim. Postures 2-5)—slam the doors shut smothering the opponent like throwing a wet blanket on top of him.

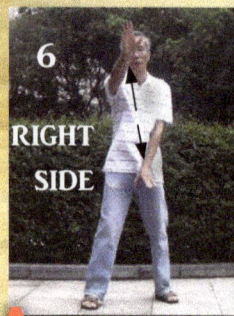 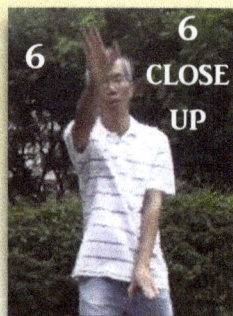 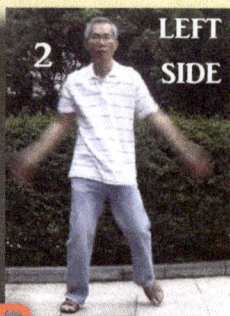

6) From 5, strike palm strikes immediately, without reservation. Visible hands strike invisible blows. Also 5) defend against a front kick and 6) palm strike

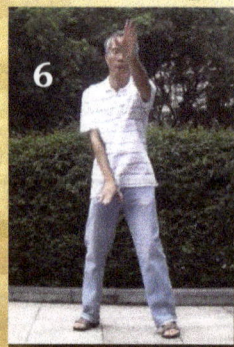 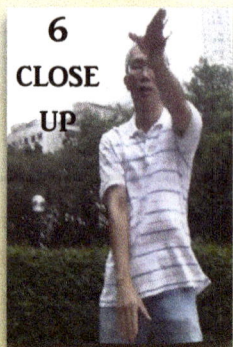

Bao Zhang, palm skills are sometimes defense or offense and sometimes defense and offense together, as above.

- Cover
- Protect
- Strike

BAO ZHANG – PALM STRIKE

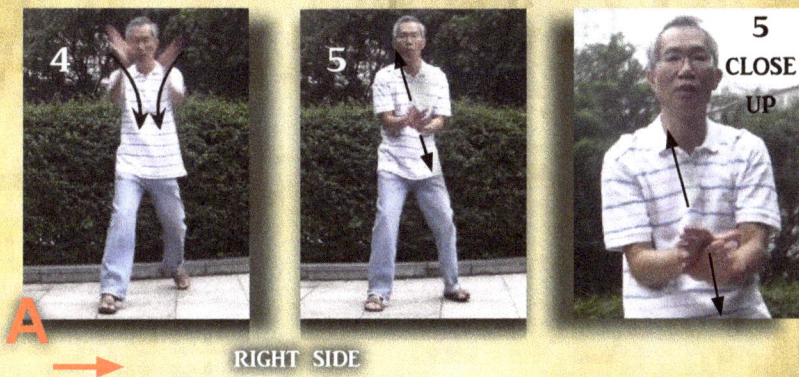

4

5

5 CLOSE UP

A →

RIGHT SIDE

2–5) PALMS COVER, PROTECT, DEFEND, SHIELD AND BIND THE OPPONENT

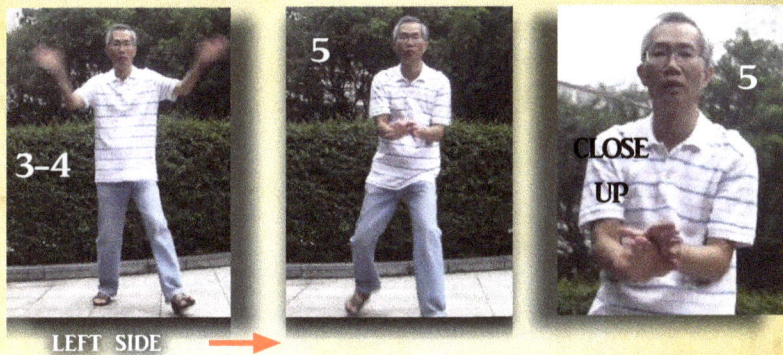

3–4

5

5 CLOSE UP

LEFT SIDE →

ALTERNATE RIGHT SIDE – LEFT SIDE 36 TIMES

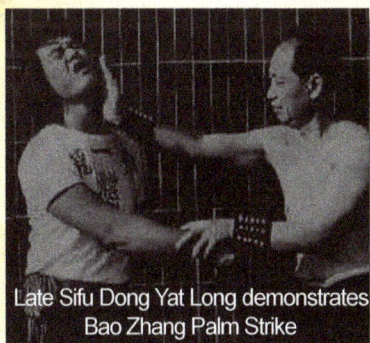

Late Sifu Dong Yat Long demonstrates
Bao Zhang Palm Strike

- Palms cover, bind, protect, defend, shield and palm strike.

- Palm attacks sometimes preceded by fingertip strikes which flatten into palm strikes.

- Against soft targets use fists.

- Against hard targets strike with the palms.

- From beggar's hand, slam the doors shut and palm strike.

53

12 BASIC SKILLS – #6 批　割　擒拿

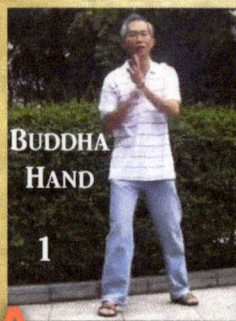 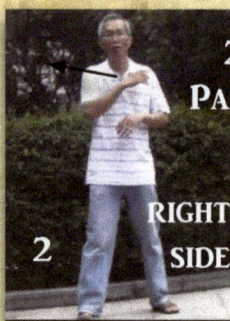 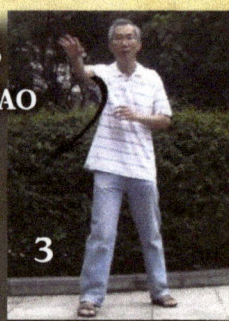

1) Buddha Hand Posture 2) Step right and 3) Pai Sao (Knife-hand strike right - edge of the palm strike) 5a) Below see the close-up image of the Qin Na Grab using Tiger Mouth grip - grab the collar bone with thumb and forefinger and rip downward.

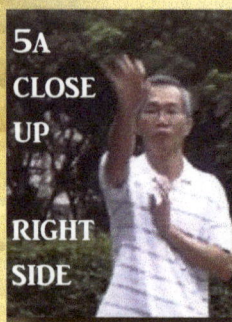 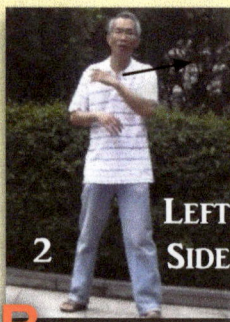 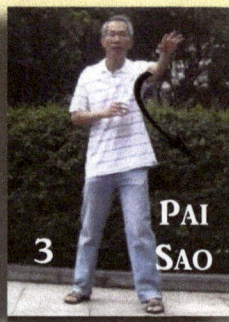

One step and three hand actions 2-5). Repeat on the left side and alternate right side and left side a minimum of thirty six times.

Pai Sao knife-edge hand is also used in USA Kwongsai Mantis' two man sets of 'Mui Hua' Plum Flower and 'Um Hon' Five Form fist. In addition, it is the 'Fic Shu' shown in the previous 'warmup' chapter.

Gwak Shu, sweeping hand, hooks and deflects the opponent's strike across the centerline down and outward covering and defending one's middle gate from solar plexus to the groin.

The traditional use of Qin Na, in this hand skill, was to rip out, using the Mantis claw, the opponent's collar bone. However, less strength is needed to rip the soft tissue of the face, throat, abdomen, etc.

PAI SAO, GWAK SAO, QIN NA

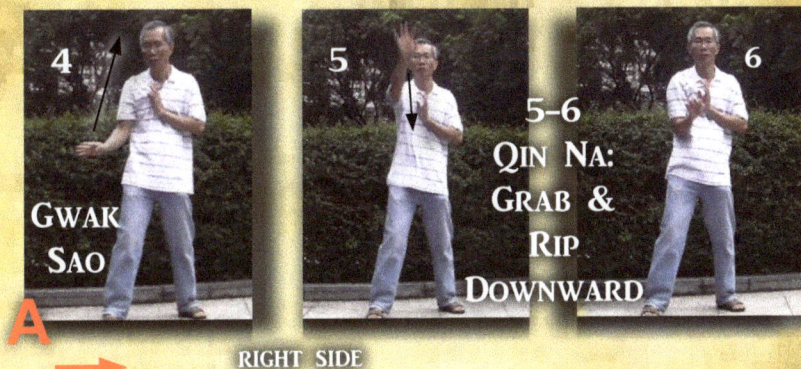

4 GWAK SAO

A →

5 5-6 QIN NA: GRAB & RIP DOWNWARD

6

RIGHT SIDE

2–5) ONE STEP (R) THREE ACTIONS
1) PAI SAO KNIFE HAND, 2) GWAK SAO SWEEPING HAND,
3) QIN NA GRAB COLLAR BONE AND RIP DOWNWARD

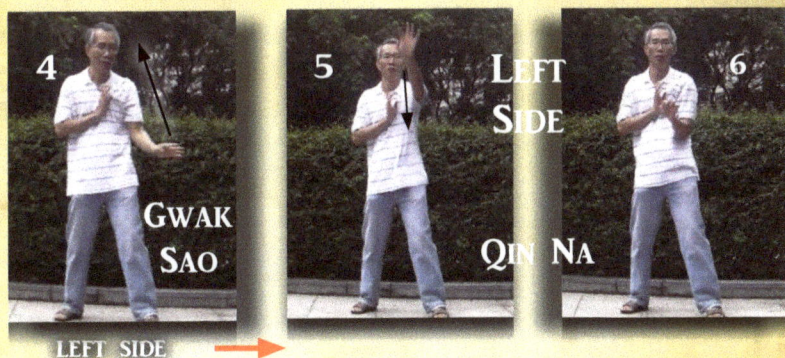

4 GWAK SAO

LEFT SIDE

5 LEFT SIDE

QIN NA

6

LEFT SIDE →

ALTERNATE RIGHT SIDE – LEFT SIDE 36 TIMES

Pai Sao knife-edge hand is similar to the "karate chop" but employs 'tan ging' elastic spring force.

Gwak Shu, sweeping hand, can be single or double bridge. Refer to my book, "Eighteen Buddha Hands" for in-depth details of the basic hand skills. This book is to illustrate the single man Chu Gar training as transmitted from Lao Sui to Chu Kai Ming.

Qin Na means to seize, trap, lock, and or break. One may tear apart an opponent's muscles or tendons, displace his joints or bones, cause strangulation (stop the opponent's breath), or interrupt the opponent's blood circulation and qi-vital energy using Qin Na.

12 BASIC SKILLS – #7 搖手 鷹擒

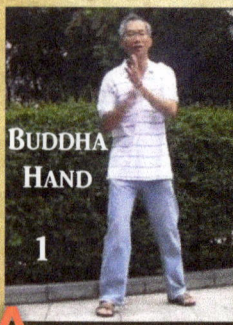

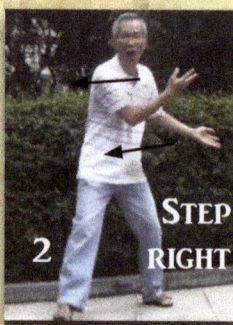

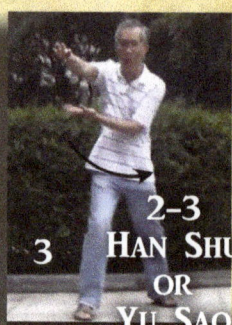

BUDDHA HAND
1

STEP RIGHT
2

2-3 HAN SHU OR YU SAO
3

RIGHT SIDE

A

1) Buddha Hand Posture 2) Step right prepare and 3) Han Shu or Yu Sao right. Han Shu (Yu Sao) is an upper right Pai Sao knife-hand strike with simultaneous left under fingertip (or phoenix fist) strike. It may also be three point: forearm deflection, Pai Sao knife-edge strike, and underneath strike.

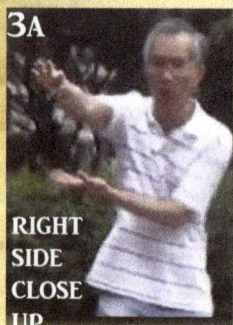

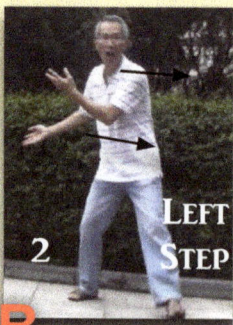

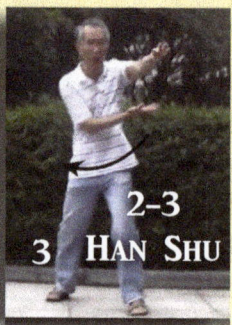

3A

RIGHT SIDE CLOSE UP

LEFT STEP
2

2-3 HAN SHU
3

LEFT SIDE

B

One step and three hand actions 2-6). 2-3) Han Shu, 4-5) Circle over grab and twist 6) pull and twist inward while punching straight jik shu strike

Yu Sao is the usually the second single man form taught in Chu Gar. Refer to my books, "Chu Gar Gao" and "Chu Gar Mantis" for details of the complete single man form "Som Gin Yu Sao." In this skill #7, Yu Sao refers to the individual hand (2-3).

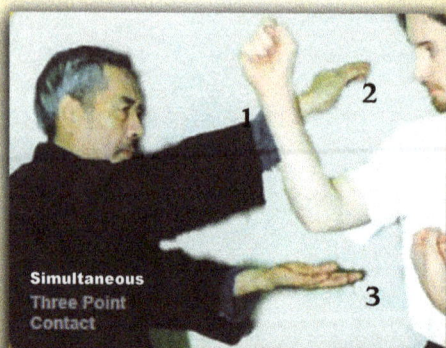

Simultaneous Three Point Contact

1 2 3

HAN SHU, CLAW–GRAB, JIK STRIKE

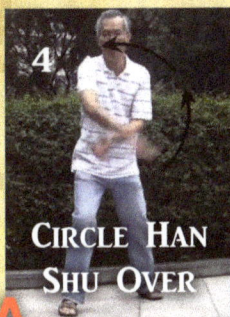

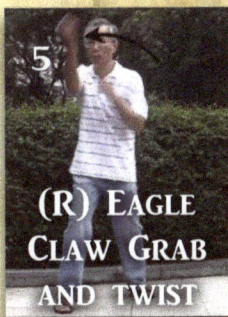

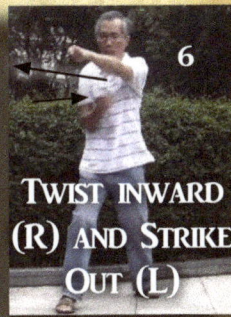

4 CIRCLE HAN SHU OVER

5 (R) EAGLE CLAW GRAB AND TWIST

6 TWIST INWARD (R) AND STRIKE OUT (L)

A →

RIGHT SIDE

2-6) ONE STEP (R) THREE ACTIONS
ONE: 2-3) HAN SHU TWO: 4-5) CIRCLE OVER GRAB AND TWIST
THREE: 6) PULL & TWIST INWARD, PHOENIX EYE STRIKE OUT

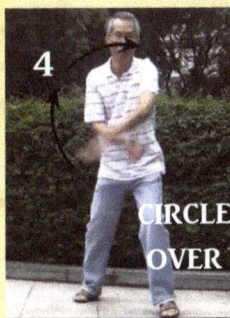

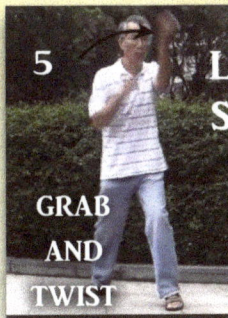

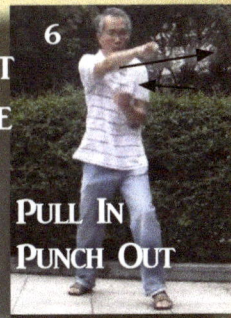

4 CIRCLE OVER

5 LEFT SIDE GRAB AND TWIST

6 PULL IN PUNCH OUT

LEFT SIDE →

ALTERNATE RIGHT SIDE – LEFT SIDE 36 TIMES

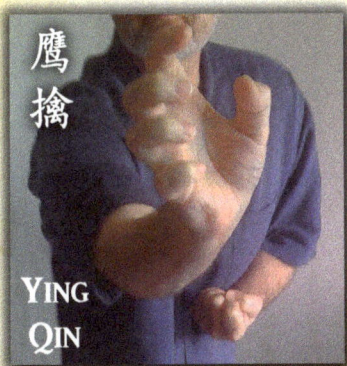

鷹擒

YING QIN

Yu Sao is called 'Han Sao or Han Shu' in USA Kwongsai Mantis and is employed in the two man sets of 'Loose Hands 1, Som Bo Gin, 108 Subset, and Um Hon Five Form fist' and the single man forms 'Um Hon, 18, and 108'.

Yu - Shake, wave, rock, turn, swing
Sao (Shu, Shou) - hand (arm)

Ying - Eagle or hawk talons
Qin - Capture, seize, or catch

57

12 Basic Skills – #8 猛单手

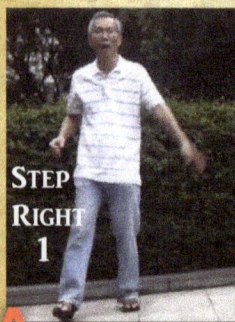

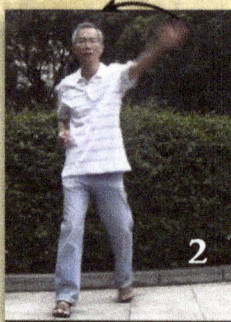

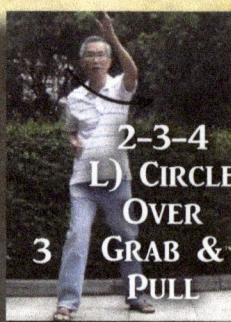

STEP RIGHT 1

2

2-3-4 L) CIRCLE OVER GRAB & PULL

3

RIGHT SIDE

A

1-4) As the opponent strikes your centerline, keeping your elbow parallel to the ground, circle over the top and grab his hand 5-6) jerk and pull backwards as you strike forward fiercely with the opposite hand. Pulling the opponent into the outgoing strike causes excess concussive force.

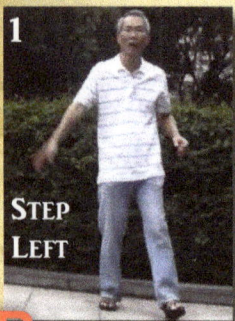

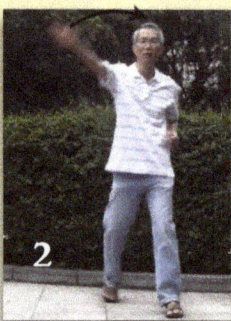

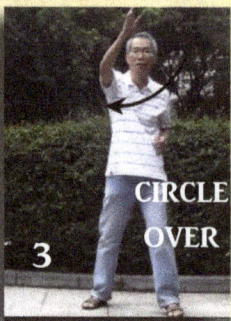

1

STEP LEFT

2

3

CIRCLE OVER

LEFT SIDE

B

As you jerk and pull the opponent forward, the opposite hand strike may be either phoenix fist or the Pai Sao knife-edge of the hand.

Mang Dan Sao shown here is the individual skill. There is also a Mang Dan Sao 'Dui Jong' or two man training routine which consists of 5 actions ending with this #8 hand skill. *Refer to my book, "Chu Gar Gao" for this 'Dui Jong' instruction.* Some Chu Gar factions end their single man forms with Mang Dan Sao before the final salute.

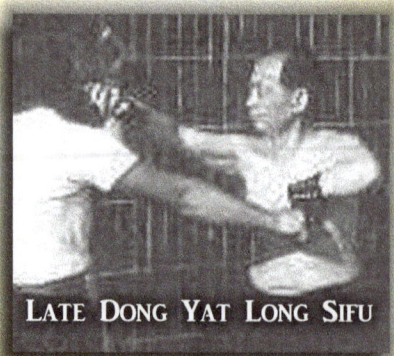

LATE DONG YAT LONG SIFU

58

Mang Dan Sao – Fierce Single Strike

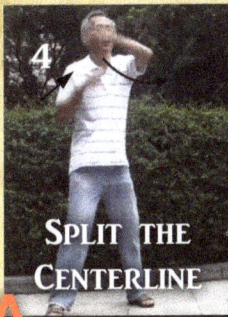

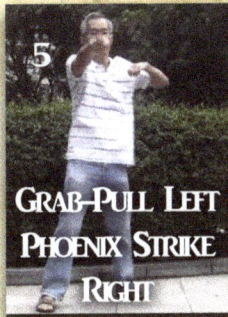

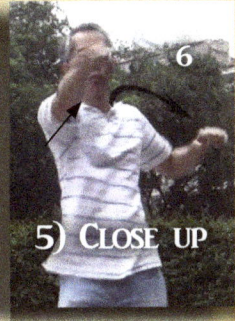

4 SPLIT THE CENTERLINE

5 GRAB–PULL LEFT PHOENIX STRIKE RIGHT

6 5) CLOSE UP

A →

RIGHT SIDE

1-6) One Step Two actions
One: 1-4) Circle Over Grab & Pull Back from Centerline
Two 5-6) Pull Back and Strike Fiercely with Opposite Hand

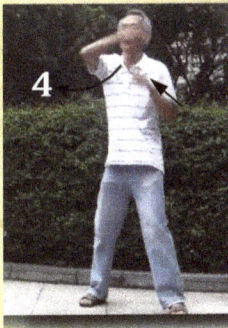

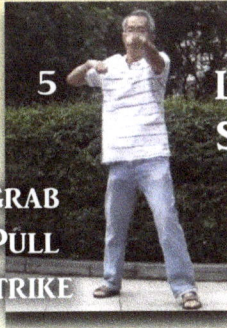

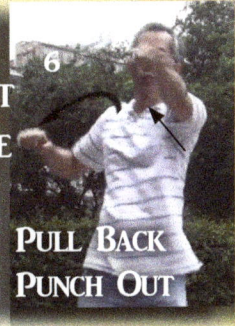

4

5 GRAB PULL STRIKE

6 LEFT SIDE — PULL BACK PUNCH OUT

LEFT SIDE →

Alternate Right Side – Left Side 36 times

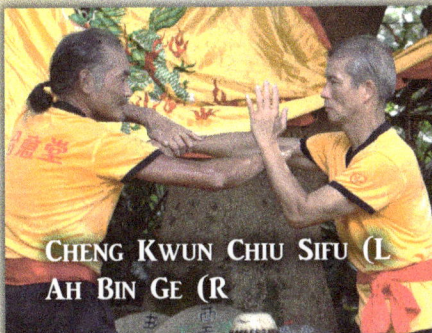

CHENG KWUN CHIU SIFU (L
AH BIN GE (R

Mang Dan Sao is found in USA Kwongsai Mantis single man form 'Um Hon Five Fist Form'.

Mang - Fierce
Dan - single, one
Sao (Shu, Shou) - hand (arm)

59

12 Basic Skills – #9 擒箭

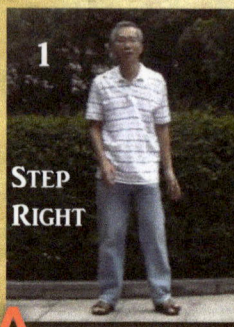

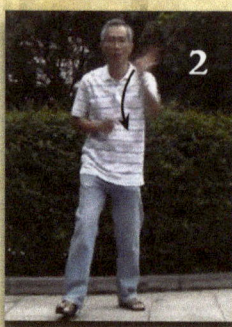

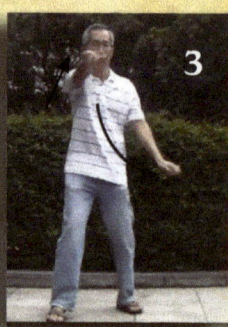

RIGHT SIDE

Qin Jian – Sweep & Straight Strike

One step and two simultaneous actions: Gwak Sao Sweeping Hand and Jik Sao Straight Phoenix Eye punch. Sweep against kicks and simultaneously strike.

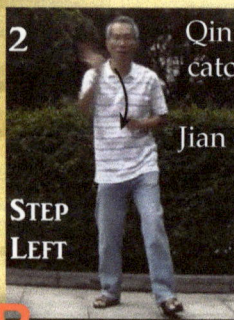

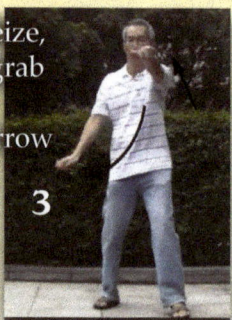

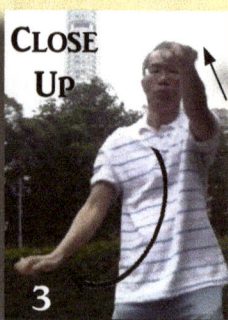

LEFT SIDE

Alternate Right Side – Left Side 36 times

This skill is used for blocking kicks. It requires a solid stance and root. It is Gwak Sao sweeping hand and simultaneous Jik Sao straight punch. Both hands shoot out at the same time. The sweeping hand is closed in a (Qin) ginger fist to avoid injuring the fingers when deflecting the opponents leg.

There is no delay - from right side, immediately step left and sweep against kicks simultaneously strike straight. Repeat alternating steps thirty six times. This is a long horse technique - lead foot and striking hand is on the same side. Short horse is the striking hand is opposite the lead foot.

12 BASIC SKILLS – #10 沈挣 抯手

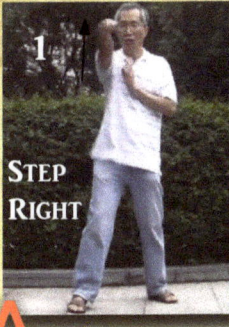 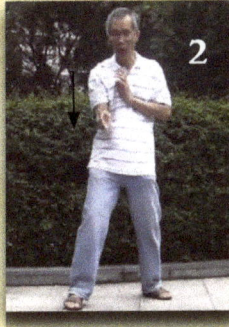 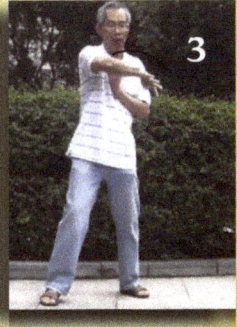

STEP RIGHT

A →

RIGHT SIDE

JIK SAO – CHUM KIU – SAI SAO

One step and 3 actions: 1) Phoenix Eye straight punch 2) Sink: drop the body center and elbow downward 3) Sai Sao: a twisting forearm deflection across centerline

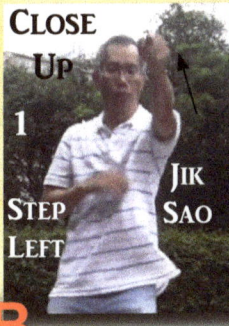 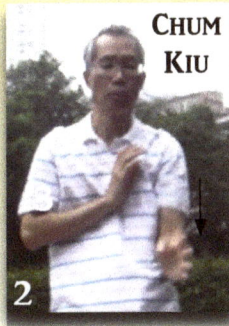 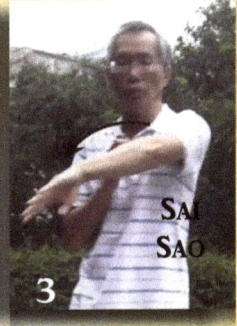

CLOSE UP

JIK SAO

STEP LEFT

CHUM KIU

SAI SAO

B →

LEFT SIDE

ALTERNATE RIGHT SIDE – LEFT SIDE 36 TIMES

Jik Sao - Phoenix Eye Straight Punch
Chum Kiu - sinking the body center and elbow down; rooting
Sai Sao (Qian) - change, flow past, yield to force

Float and sink (Chum Kiu) are two important principles. Float is the sudden release of force, explosive energy. Sink is more difficult to master because it depends on one's natural ability to learn "feeling" or perceive the opponent's exertion of force. He who has mastered this is capable of rendering his opponent completely immobile, thus putting him under absolute control. When the opponent moves, one simply sinks the center into him.

61

12 Basic Skills – #11 角捶 带手 极掌

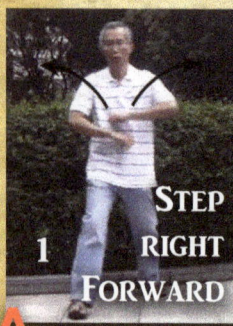
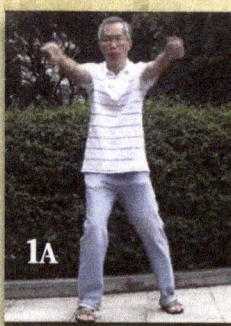
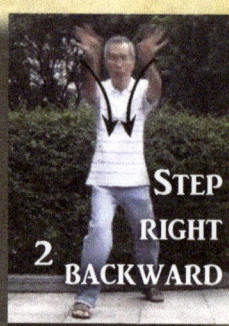

RIGHT SIDE

This Hand Skill #11 is known as 蓋打 包桩 **Kup Da Bao Zhang.** It is similar to Hand #5. Simply stated it teaches breaking free, stepping forward and back, and slamming the doors shut with an extreme palm strike. 蓋 Kup (Gai) - cover, lid, cap, put a cover on top; 打 Da - strike, hit, knock, break, smash,beat,fight,attack; 包 Bao - cover, protect, shield, wrap around; 桩 Zhuang - stake, pile, wooden post

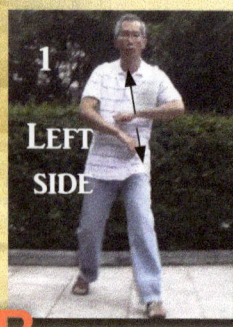
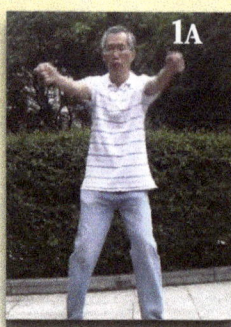
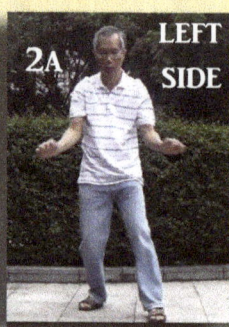

1A) 角 Jiao 捶 Chui - hammer fist in the shape of ox horns, 2A) 带 Dai 手 Sao - take, bring, or carry the opponent's hands, 3A) 极 Ji 掌 Zhang - utmost strike with the palm

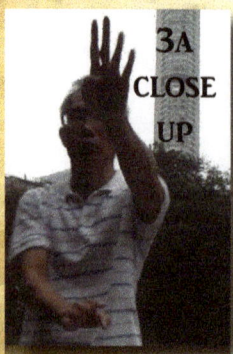

This **Hand #11** is used to break the grab of an opponent, like a judo lapel grab. But it also trains footwork. Advance, retreat, and advance again - forward, back, forward. Dui Jong two man uses this footwork. It also shows the four principles: float, sink, swallow, spit. 1A) Gow Choy is float and spit. 2A) Dai Shou is sink and swallow. 3A) Bao Zhang is spit.

BAO ZHANG – PALM STRIKE

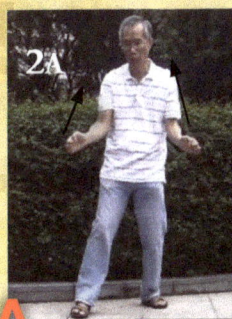

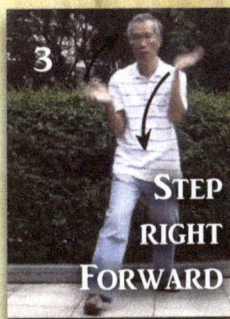

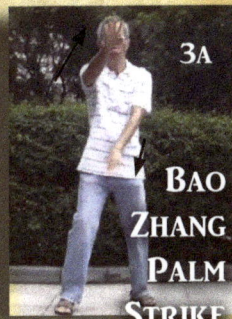

2A

3

**STEP
RIGHT
FORWARD**

3A

**BAO
ZHANG
PALM
STRIKE**

A →   RIGHT SIDE

2–5) PALMS COVER, PROTECT, DEFEND, SHIELD AND BIND THE OPPONENT

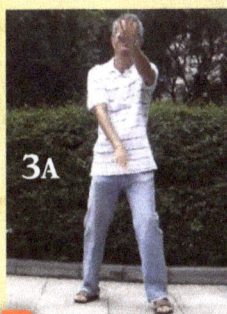

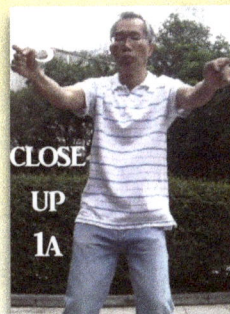

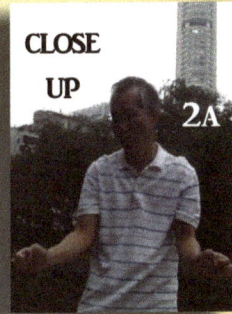

3A

**CLOSE
UP
1A**

**CLOSE
UP**

2A

B LEFT SIDE →

ALTERNATE RIGHT SIDE – LEFT SIDE 36 TIMES

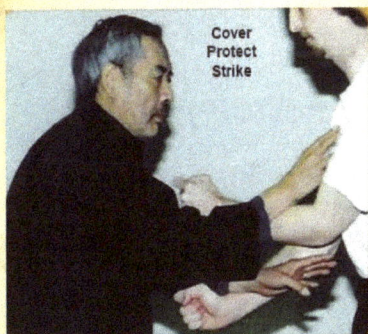

Cover
Protect
Strike

Late Sifu Louie Jack Man - Bao Zhang

The Bao Zhang **Hand Skill #5** uses the palm heel strike. Fingers pointing slightly outward is the correct posture. This Bao Zhang **Hand #11** uses the whole palm and strikes the face, nose, eyes and soft tissue.

- Cover
- Protect
- Strike

63

12 Basic Skills #12 批挣 极挣 连底挣

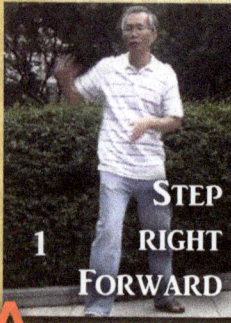
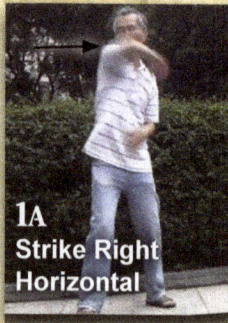
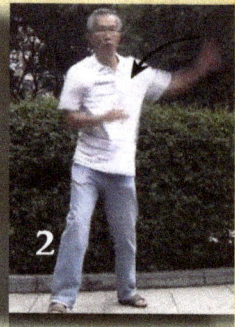

A →

RIGHT SIDE →

Jang Shu, elbow strokes may be employed as defense and offense. Sticky elbow methods are many and varied and contained in the two man forms. It is said, " You can prevent your opponent from defeating you through defense, but you cannot defeat him without taking the offensive."

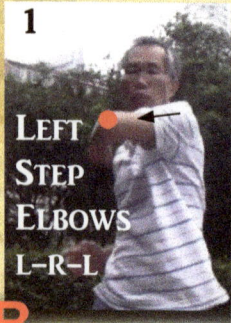
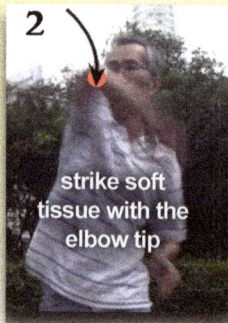
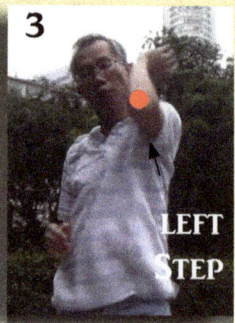

B →

LEFT SIDE →

One step and three alternating elbow strikes changing arms each strike. Step right and strike right, left, right elbows. Step left and strike left, right, left elbows; horizontal, over, under.

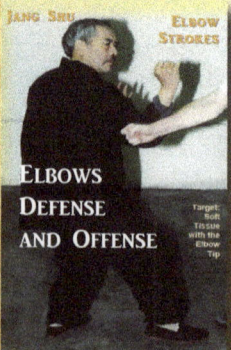

- 10 Elbow Strokes is a basic Kwongsai Mantis exercise: Forward, right, left, 90 degree turns, and return step
- Photo right—segmented power— second hand elbow stroke turns to first hand fingertip strike.
- Continuous alternating horizontal elbow strokes.
- Primarily single bridge striking; Inside or outside the bridge.

JANG SHU – (3) ELBOW STROKES

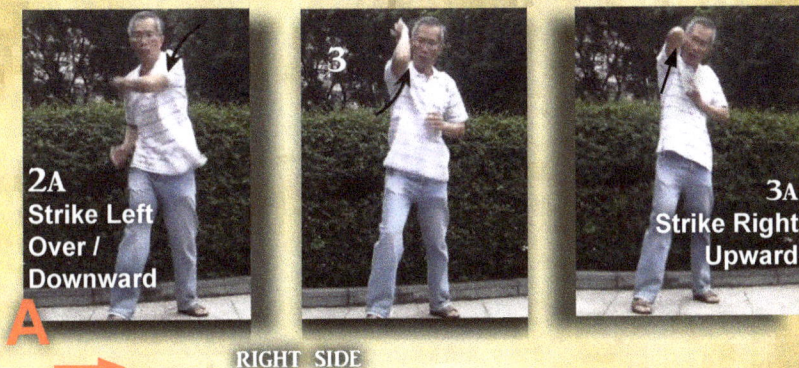

2A
**Strike Left
Over /
Downward**

3

3A
**Strike Right
Upward**

A

RIGHT SIDE

ONE STEP & THREE ELBOW STRIKES – HORIZONTAL, DOWNWARD, & UPWARD STRIKE
ONE STEP – EACH ELBOW STRIKE CHANGE ARMS

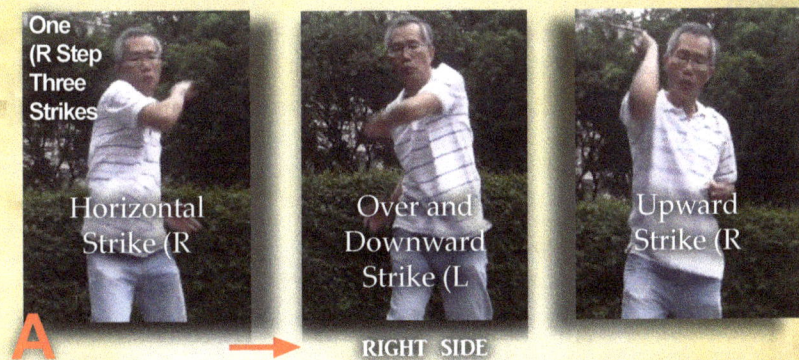

One
(R Step
Three
Strikes

Horizontal
Strike (R

Over and
Downward
Strike (L

Upward
Strike (R

A

RIGHT SIDE

ALTERNATE 36 TIMES RIGHT SIDE 3 STROKES – LEFT SIDE 3 STROKES

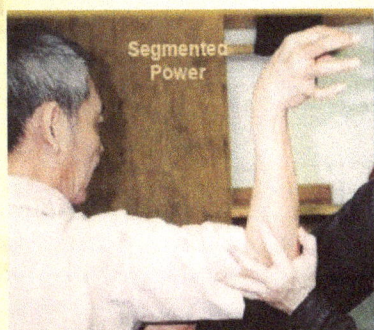

Segmented
Power

Late Sifu Louie Jack Man - Elbow Sroke

Segmented power - the Mantis arm has three hands: Shoulder, elbow, wrist to fingertips. If the second hand elbow stroke is blocked one may simply segment the next hand and strike with the first hand fist, palm, or fingertips.

- 3 Continuous Elbow Strokes
- Right Side (R, L, R)
- Left Side (L, R, L)
- 3 - Horizontal, Over, Under 65

12 BASIC SKILLS GLOSSARY

Refer to my book "Eighteen Buddha Hands" for details of hands listed in red. The Chinese characters and Pinyin names in black are those of Chan Sifu. See the Appendix: Note on Hand Names & Translations.

1 绞 **Gow Choy**
绞 Jiao (3rd tone Mandarin) - twist, wring, entangle, ream, wind up
    strike as a meat mincer, continuous Hammer Fist Strikes

2 将 抖 押 **Jik, Mor, Bil, Gop, Jik, Narp, Chop**
       将   (Lu) Luo (1st) rub, push, smooth out,
        stroke the tiger's whiskers (Mor Sao)
        strip a twig of its leaves
       Luo - Mor Sao - wax on, wax off,

    抖 Dou (3rd) tremble, shiver, quiver, shake, jerk, vibrate
        Pluck up one's spirits
        Spread the quilt with a flick
        Shake the snow off one's clothes
        Give the reins a jerk
        Bil Jee - Gop Sao - Jik Sao

      押 Ya (1st) security, detain, take into custody
        Narp Sao - Chun Sao

3 拈挣 传手 背剑 **Jik, Mor, Bil, Gop, Jik, Narp, Chop Sao**
   拈 Nian (1st) pick up with the thumb and one or two fingers
        take candy from a jar
     挣 Zheng (1st) struggle, struggle for existence
Nian Zheng - capture and twist the opponent's arm with tiger's
        mouth (Fu Kou) grip

       传 Chuan (2nd) pass, pass off
        Passoff to someone else
     手 Sao, Shu, Shou (3rd) - hand or arm
Chuan Sao - pass off from one hand to another

        背剑 Bei Jian
   背 Bei (4th) back of the body, back of an object
      剑 Jian (4th) sword or sabre
Bei Jian - power from the back, hand as sword

12 BASIC SKILLS GLOSSARY

4   格   Choc Sao - Jik Sao

Ge (2nd) impede, obstruct, bar from, fight,
Ge Dou (2nd-4th) grapple, wrestle, fight, fight with bare fists, fistfight
Choc Sao - Jik Sao

5   包桩 Bao Zhuang Palm Strike

包 Bao (1st) cover, protect, shield, wrap around
桩 Zhuang (1st) stake, pile, wooden post
Bao Zhuang - cover the opponent (zhuang) and strike with palm

6   批 割 擒拿 Pai Sao, Gwak Sao, Qin Na

批 Pi (1st) slap, cut into slices with the edge of the hand
割 Ge (1st) cut off, remove, excise, mow the grass, sweep or cut to the side
Qin Na 擒拿 Qin (2nd) capture, seize, catch Na (2nd) take hold, firm grasp

7   摇手 鹰擒 Han Shu, Claw-Grab, Jik Straight Strike

Yao Shou, Yu Sao 摇手
摇 Yao (2nd) shake, wave, rock, turn, sway, swing
手 Sao, Shu, or Shou (3rd) hand or arm

Ying Qin 鹰擒
鹰 Ying (1st) eagle or hawk talons
擒 Qin (2nd) capture, seize, catch

8   Mang Dan Sao 猛单手 - Fierce Single Strike

猛 Mang (3rd) fierce, violent, energetic, vigorous
单 Dan (1st) one, single, solitary
手 Sao, Shu, Shou (3rd) hand or arm

9   Qin Jian 擒箭 - Sweep Away and Straight Strike

擒 Qin (2nd) capture, seize, catch
箭 Jian (4th) arrow shot from a bow
* (Jian Bu) A sudden big stride forward (USA Kwongsai Mantis)
* (San Bu Jian) Three Step Arrow

10   沈挣 揷手 Jik Sao, Chum Kiu, Sai Sao

沈挣 Chen Zheng (Chum Kiu)
沈 Chen (2nd) sink, sink down, lower down, feel heavy

12 BASIC SKILLS GLOSSARY

10 Cont'd: 沈挣 摡手 Jik Sao, Chum Kiu, Sai Sao
挣 Zheng (1st) struggle
*Float, Sink, Swallow, Spit four word secret: Sink=Chum

摡手 Sai Sao
摡 Sai (Qian) (1st) change, yield to, flow past, roll over
手 Sao, Shu, Shou (3rd) hand or arm

11 角捶 带手 极掌 - Jiao Chui, Dai Shou, Bao Zhang
角 Jiao (3rd) - in the shape of ox horns
捶 Chui (4th) - beat with fist, thump, pound, bang, hammer

带 Dai (4th) take, bring, or carry the opponent's hand
手 Sao, Shu, Shou (3rd) hand or arm

极 Ji (2nd) extreme, greatest extent, utmost
掌 Zhang (3rd) palm, strike with the palm, slap

*蓋打 包桩 Kup Da Bao Zhang
蓋 Kup (Gai) (4th) cover, lid, cap, put a cover on top
打 Da (3rd) strike, hit, knock, break, smash, beat, fight, attack
包 Bao (1st) cover, protect, shield, wrap around
桩 Zhuang (1st) stake, pile, wooden post

12 批挣 极挣 连底挣 - Pi Zheng,Ji Zheng, Liandi Zheng-**3 Elbows**

批 Pi (1st) slap, cut into slices with the edge of the hand
挣 Zheng (1st) struggle

极 Ji (2nd) extreme, greatest extent, utmost
挣 Zheng (1st) struggle

连 Lian (2nd) link, join, connect, one after another, continuous, in
succession, circular
底 Di (3rd) bottom, base, end up with, come to
挣 Zheng (1st) struggle
*There are 4 tones in spoken Mandarin.
The inflection is listed after the name.

SEQUENTIAL TRANSMISSION

Step by step, if you have been following the sequential transmission of late Chu Kai Ming Sifu's teaching, you have trained now:

- Warmups

- Horse Steps

- Hard Bridge Som Bo Gin - Sun Yu Hing's teaching

- Hard Bridge Som Bo Gin - Chu Kai Ming's teaching (only Line Three is different)

- 12 Basic Hand Skills

    After training the 12 Hand Skills to completion one would also train, in Chu Kai Ming's transmission:

Continued Single Man Form Training

- Tan Zhuang - Soft Bridge Som Bo Gin

- Som Gin Yu Sao - Three Shaking Bridges (not taught in later days)

- 2nd Form - An advanced skill of Chu Kai Ming's Transmission

Read on now to learn of the
Tan Zhuang - Soft Bridge Som Bo Gin shadowboxing.

69

弹桩

TAN ZHUANG
ELASTIC SPRING POWER FORM

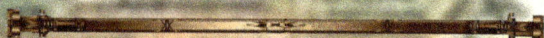

Soft Bridge Som Bo Gin

Two man training is to know others.
Single man shadowboxing is to
know one's self.

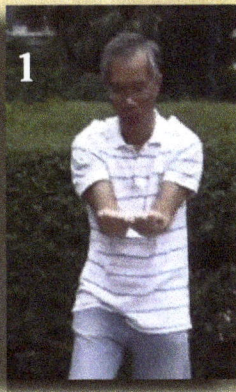

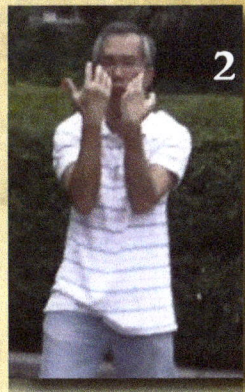

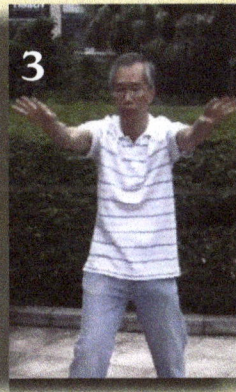

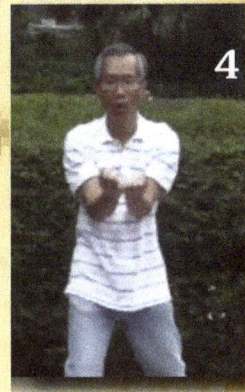

Step forward, relax & flick the hands up and out (1-4)

Relax, Relax, Completely Relax

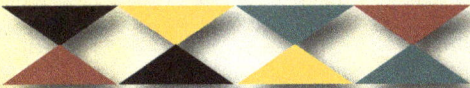

Soft Bridge Som Bo Gin Creates Gan Tan Ging

This form is found in the first generation Lao Sui teaching and as shown herein, was transmitted by late Sifu Chu Kai Ming. The form sequence is the same as the previous Hard Bridge Som Bo Gin except the emphasis is on soft elastic spring force and the 3 Arrow Steps are replaced by flicking the hands (Ping Shu) as shown in the photos above.

One should be totally relaxed. Before flicking out the Tan Zhuang spring power, pause for a moment then suddenly strike out. This will generate the 驚弹劲 Gan Tan Ging elastic spring force.

SOM BO GIN FORM—SOFT BRIDGE

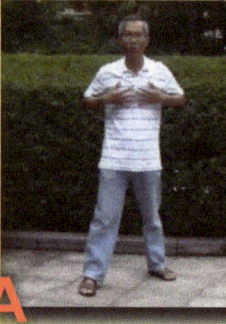

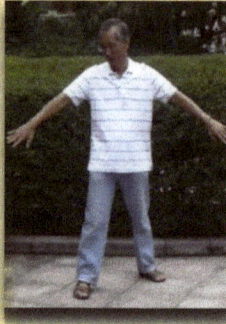

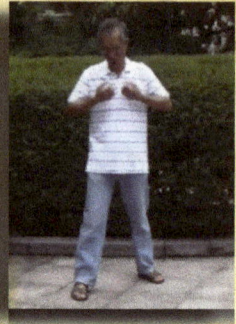

opening sequence - hand to hand - heart to heart

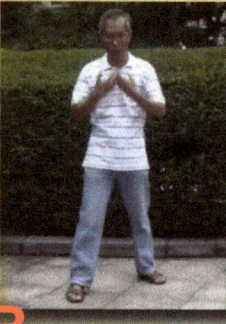

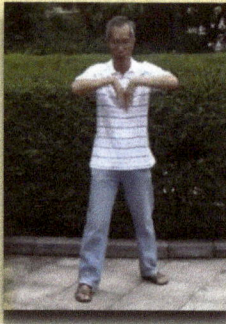

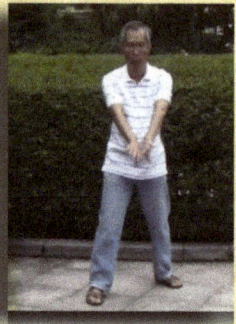

open and close - muscle tendon change

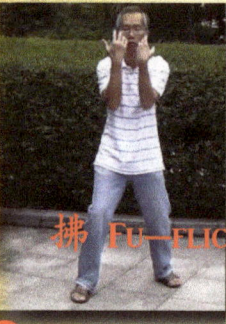

拂 FU—FLICK OUT BRISKLY

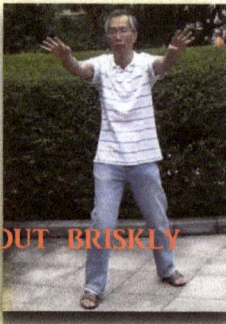

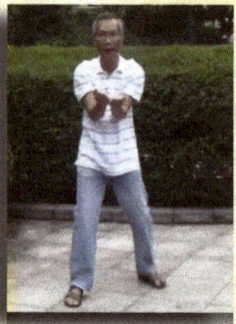

first three step - hands toward face (look in mirror), flick spring power, gop shu

TAN ZHUANG—SPRING POWER FORM

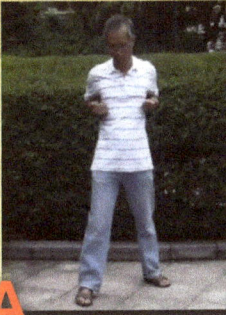

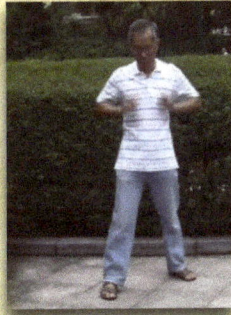

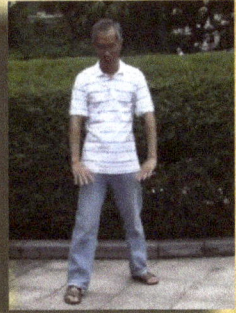

raise the stomach - compress the ribs - round the back

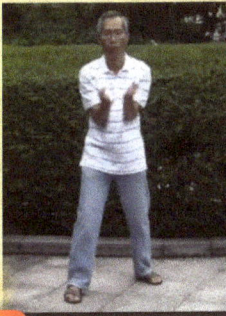

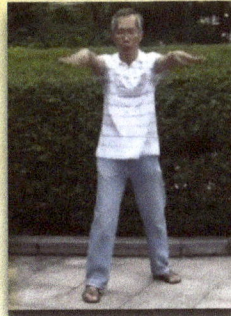

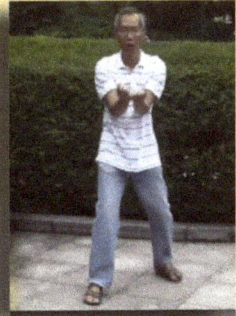

elbows inward - bil jee - gop shu

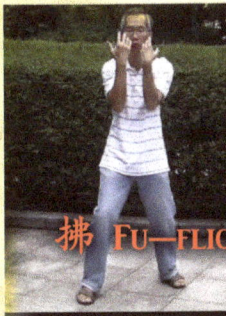

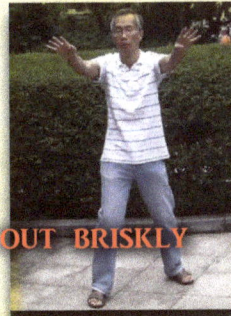

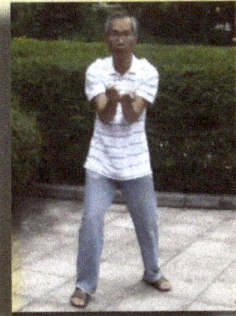

拂 FU—FLICK OUT BRISKLY

second three step - hands toward face (look in mirror), flick spring power, gop shu

SOM BO GIN FORM—SOFT BRIDGE

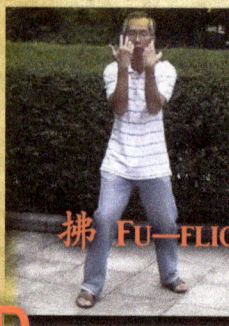

拂 FU—FLICK OUT BRISKLY

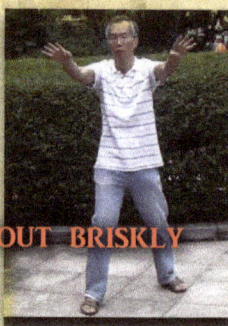

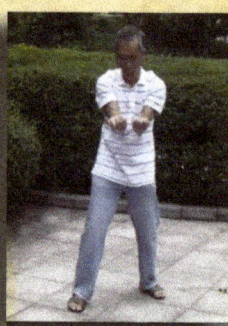

D →　　　　　　　　　　　　　　　　→

third three step - hands toward face (look in mirror), flick spring power, gop shu

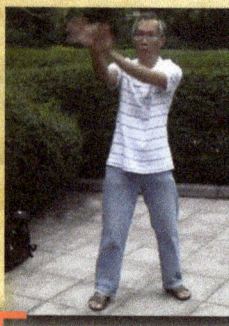

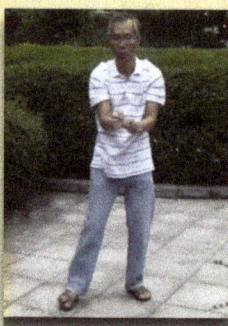

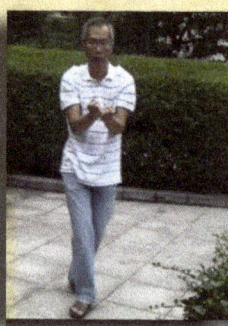

E →　　　　　　　　　　　　　　　　→

claw to gop shu - cross step to left

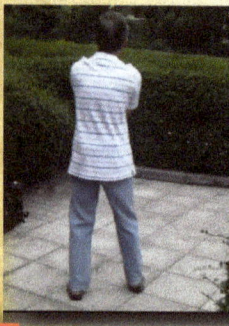

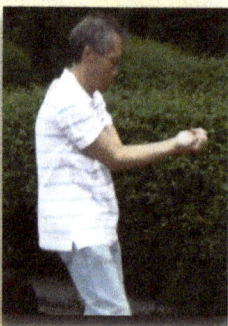

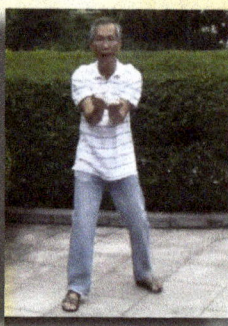

F →　　　　　　　　　　　　　　　　→

LINE TWO BEGINS - complete turn around with gop shu

74

TAN ZHUANG—SPRING POWER FORM

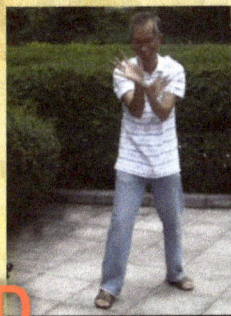

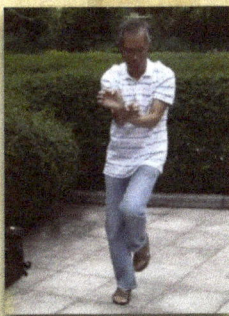

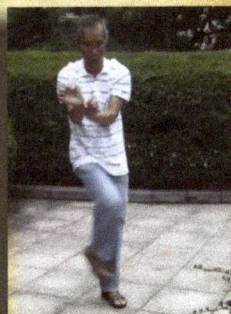

D

double claw - left, right chop steps

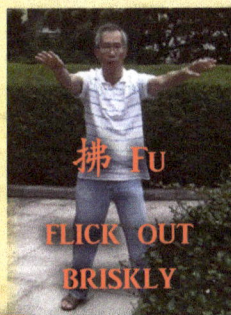

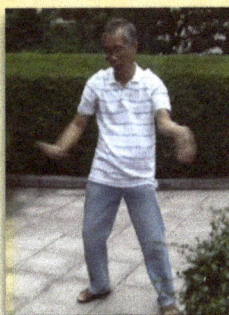

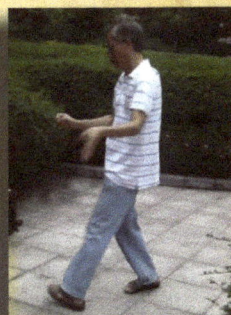

拂 Fu

FLICK OUT

BRISKLY

E

left foot - flick spring power out - turn around with locking hands

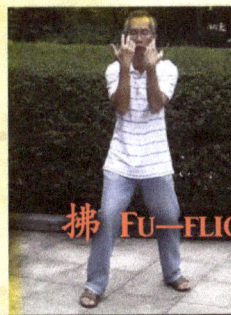

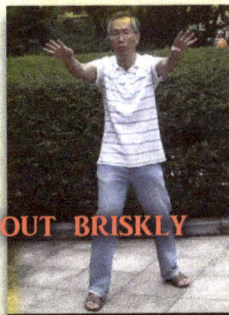

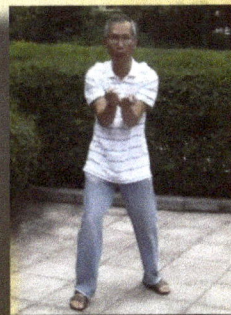

拂 Fu—FLICK OUT BRISKLY

F

SECOND LINE - first three step - hands toward face (look in mirror),
flick spring power, gop shu

Som Bo Gin Form—Soft Bridge

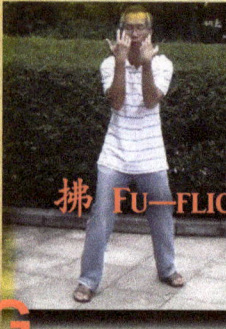

拂 **Fu—flick out briskly**

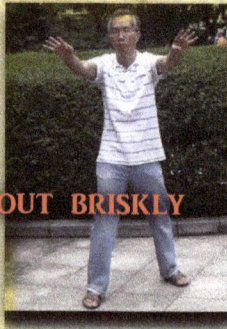

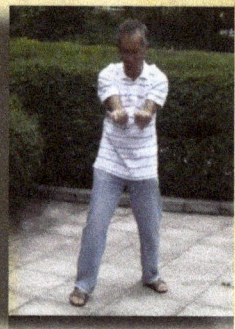

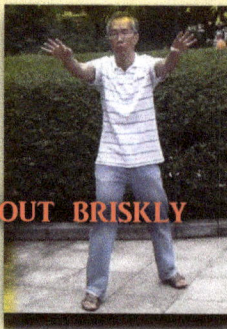

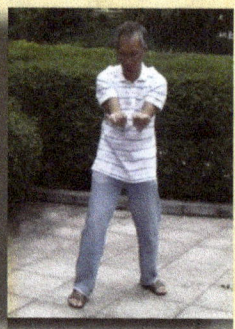

G

SECOND LINE - 2nd three step - hands toward face (look in mirror),
flick spring power, gop shu

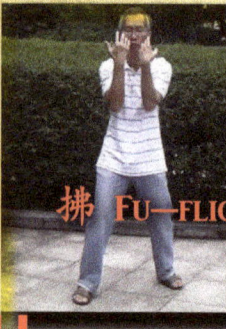

拂 **Fu—flick out briskly**

H

SECOND LINE - 4th three step - jik straight strikes, bil jee finger strikes, gop shu

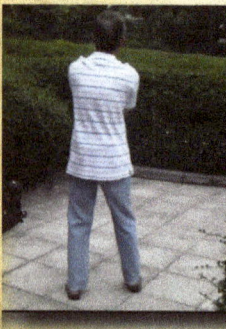

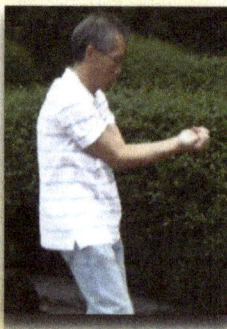

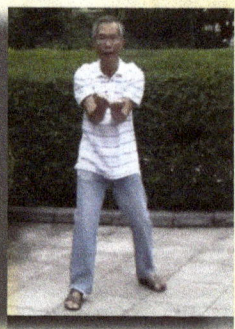

I

LINE THREE - CLOSING FORM BEGINS - complete turn around with gop shu

TAN ZHUANG—SPRING POWER FORM

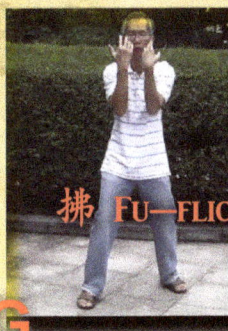

拂 Fu—FLICK OUT BRISKLY

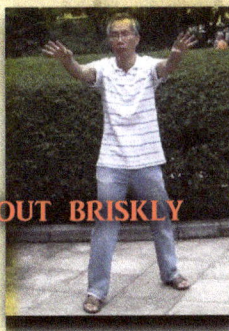

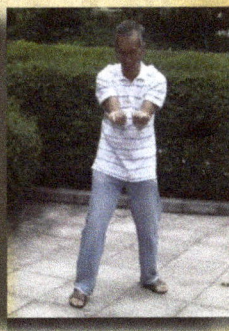

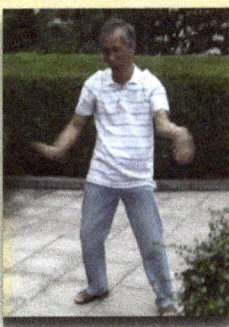

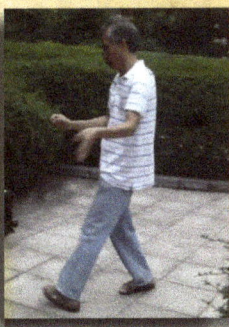

G

SECOND LINE - 3rd three step - hands toward face (look in mirror), flick spring power, gop shu

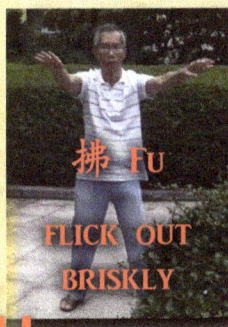

拂 Fu

FLICK OUT

BRISKLY

H

SECOND LINE - left step up - flick spring power out - turn around with locking hands

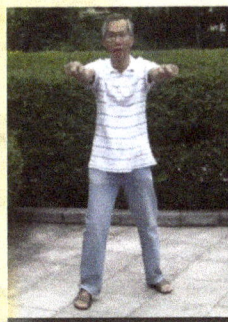

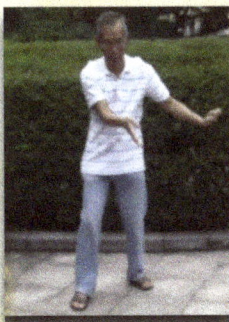

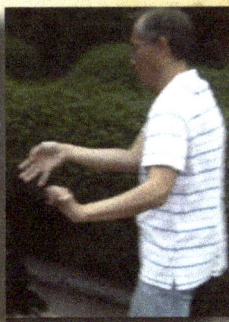

I

THIRD LINE - jik straight strikes, step back with locking hands

SOM BO GIN FORM—SOFT BRIDGE

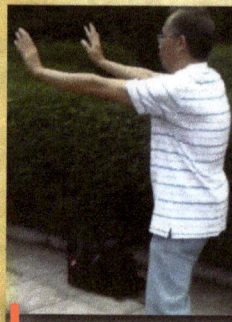

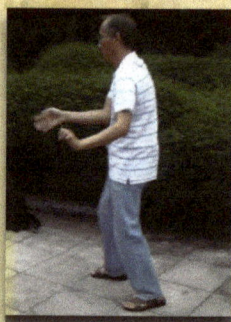

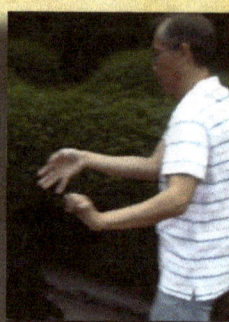

J →　　　　　　　　　　　　　　　　　　　　　　　　→

THIRD LINE - step (R) forward double palm strikes - step back with locking hands

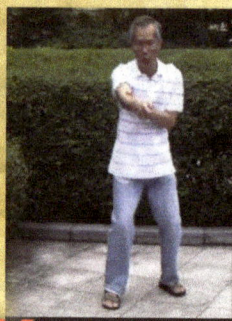

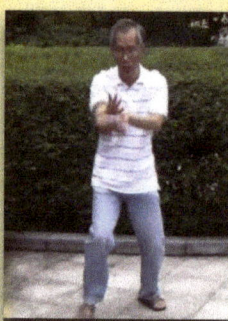

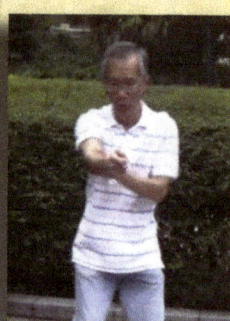

K →　　　　　　　　　　　　　　　　　　　　　　　　→

THIRD LINE - step (R) forward jik shu straight strike - repeat a second time

Tan Ging, or spring power, is likened to a "frightened reaction" - it is an automatic instinctual response. When one touches a burning stove, the hand immediately and quickly jerks away. When sensitivity is refined the 12 basic hand skills will react automatically when engaging the opponent.

Some say the beginning and the end of Southern Praying Mantis is the Som Bo Gin single man form - hard bridge and soft bridge. The meaning of this is the shadowboxing form embodies the principles and contains the fundamental skills which enable one to build a rock solid foundation.

In turn, the beginning and the end of the Som Bo Gin form is proper Mantis body posture and stance. Correct horse stance is the father of power. Mor Sao, the grinding hand, is the mother of Mantis hands.

TAN ZHUANG—SPRING POWER FORM

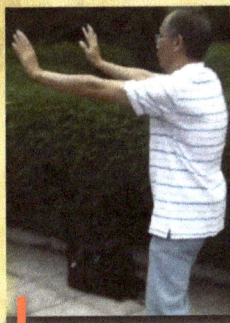

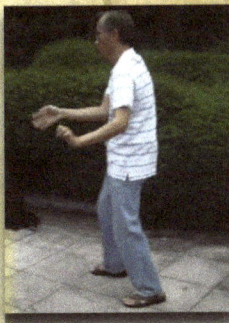

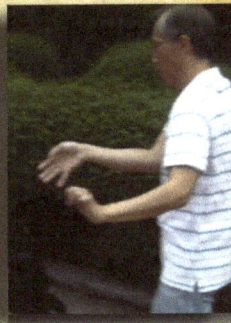

J

THIRD LINE - step (R) forward double palm strikes - step back with locking hand

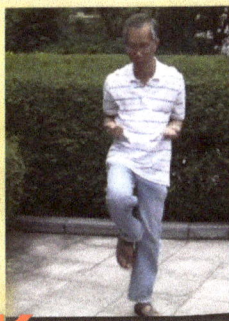

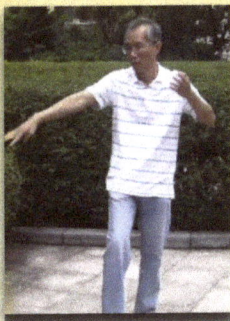

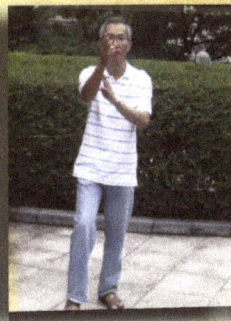

K

THIRD LINE - knee up elbows back - pai shu side - ending salute
(single bridge Hat Yi Sao Beggar's Hand right)

Power is generated through the feet and up the legs and back, and expressed in the hands. Without a firm stance there is no root and without a root there will be little power in the hands. A common saying is, "When the stance is rooted one is as immovable as Mt. Tai."

Som Bo Gin is nothing mysterious. You can say the distance of a cow lying down, fists fly with the speed of arrows, combat should begin and end within three steps and other metaphors, but the meaning is very simple; Som Bo Gin refers to three fronts of defense–up, down, and middle (shung-har-jung) and left, right, and center (zuo, you, qian). Three steps forward with three fronts of defense. The secret of Som Bo Gin is repetition of the forms, single and two man, uninterrupted over a long period of time.

Read on now for 1st generation anecdotes and details about Lao Sui's 2nd form, Som Gin Yu Kiu, followed by Chu Kai Ming's 2nd Shadowboxing form.

YANG CLAN CHU GAR IN CHINA

Yang Clan Chu Gar Mantis, descends from Yang Shou, a first generation disciple of Lao Sui, in 1920s/30s Hong Kong. Chu Kai Ming's transmission, subject of this book, is also first generation Lao Sui's teaching in Hong Kong.

They share much in common including "Tan Zhuang" Spring Power and the end sequence of Som Bo Gin, which differs in the second and succeeding generations of Chu Gar. Yip Sui and his "Chow Gar" was a second generation student of Lao Sui.

For more details of the Yang Clan and the first generation Chu Gar transmission, refer to my book shown below - available at Amazon, Barnes and Noble, Books-A-Million and other fine online retailers.

RELEASE DATE: JULY, 2015

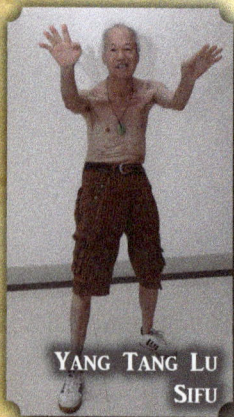

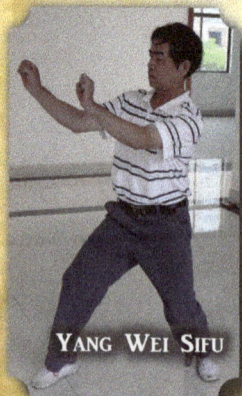

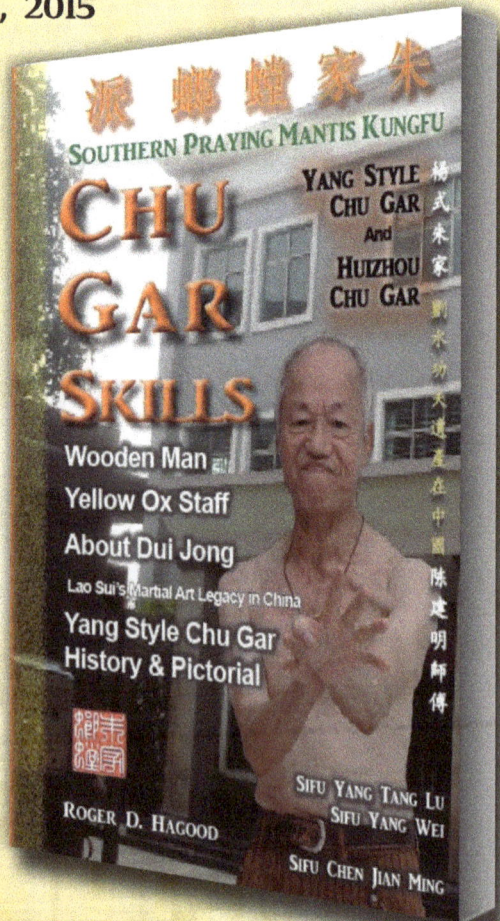

YANG TANG LU
SIFU

朱家螳螂派
SOUTHERN PRAYING MANTIS KUNGFU

CHU GAR SKILLS

YANG STYLE CHU GAR AND HUIZHOU CHU GAR

Wooden Man
Yellow Ox Staff
About Dui Jong

Lao Sui's Martial Art Legacy in China

Yang Style Chu Gar
History & Pictorial

ROGER D. HAGOOD

SIFU YANG TANG LU
SIFU YANG WEI
SIFU CHEN JIAN MING

YANG WEI SIFU

Som Gin Yu Kiu Form

Som Gin Yu Kiu, Three Steps Shaking Bridge, was the second form taught by Lao Sui. Chu Kai Ming, Lao's student, stopped teaching this at one point and taught **his own 2nd form that follows on the next page**. My two books shown below illustrate the complete Som Gin Yu Kiu form.

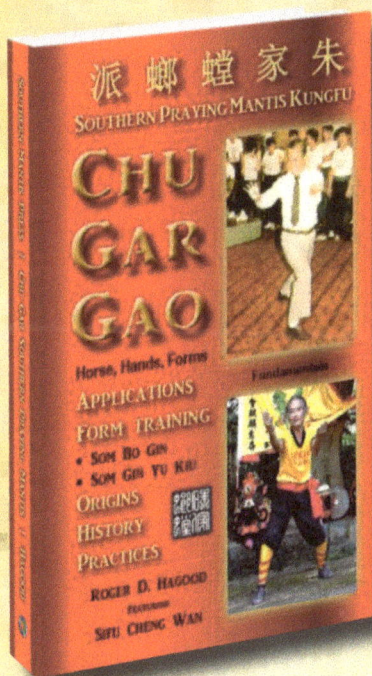

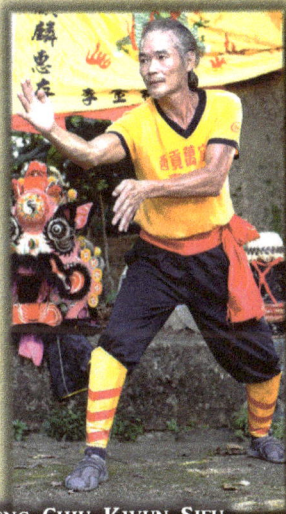

CHENG CHIU KWUN SIFU

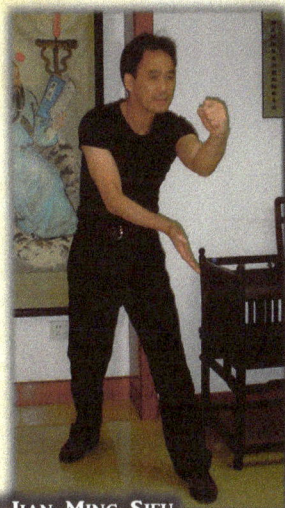

CHEN JIAN MING SIFU

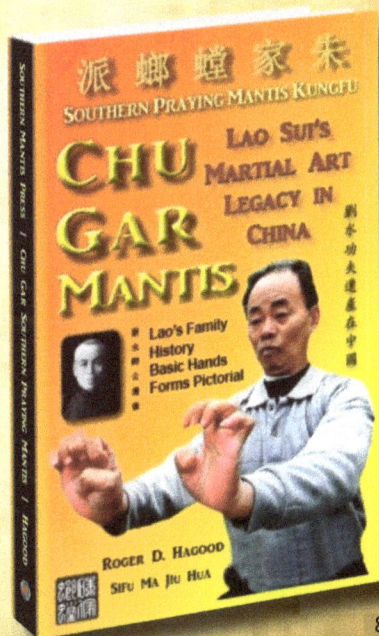

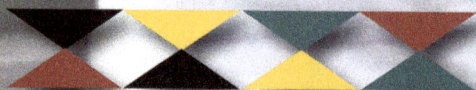

Chu Kai Ming's
Second Form

Essence of the 12 Basic Skills

無搖手不成朱家，無螳螂不成功架

Chu Gar emphasizes Yu Kiu (Shaking Bridge)
Hand techniques 'are' the Mantis postures

Mantis Shape Through Form Training

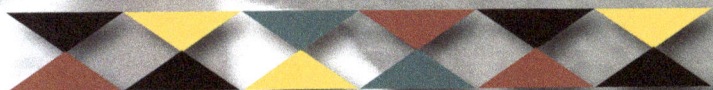

Basic Hands Linked Into Form For Solo Practice

Although Hakka Mantis combat is only mastered by two man (paired training), the essential skills must be thoroughly trained and made one's own through solo training. One must individually set a personal schedule and exercise himself daily until the fundamental skills, footwork, basic hand skills, and single man forms are instinctually understood. Follow the step by step outline in this book.

From Chan Sifu: This is a form my Sifu, Chu Kai Ming, created. I don't know if he taught the form to any other students. It may not have been his final design. I left Hong Kong in 1976 and came back in 1981. Upon return, I went to Botany garden in Central where he usually practiced his kung fu in the morning and I showed him the form again. He was kind of surprised that I still remembered it.

That showed me that he probably didn't show it to other students, or other students simply ignored it. The form is useful to recall and train the 12 basic hand techniques we learned. It has 4 lines or sections followed by the end or closing which is the same as Som Bo Gin form. The 1st line is defending attacks from the outer door. 2nd line is defending attacks on the center line. 3rd line is Yu Kiu but we didn't practice the Yu Kiu Shaking Bridge form, only the hand Yu Kiu technique and combinations. Chu Sifu previously taught Lao Sui's Yu Kiu form but had stopped teaching it when I was learning this form. The 4th section is double hand techniques, both hands attack and defend simultaneously. The closing sequence is a trademark of my Sifu, he was an expert on 绞搥 Hammer Fist.

CHU KAI MING—2ND FORM

OPENING SEQUENCE 1A - 1L

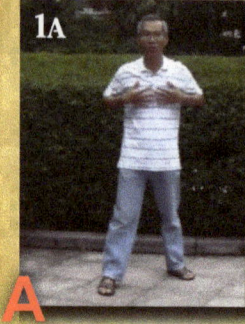

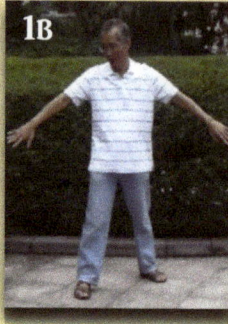

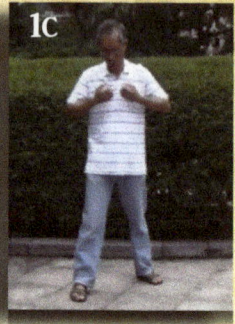

A →

opening sequence - hand to hand - heart to heart

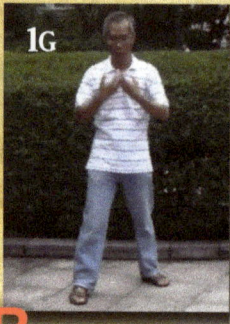

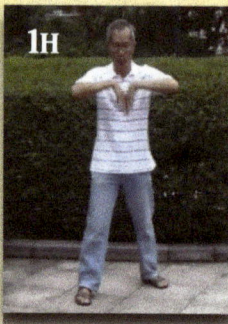

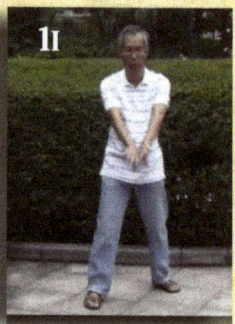

B →

open and close - muscle tendon change

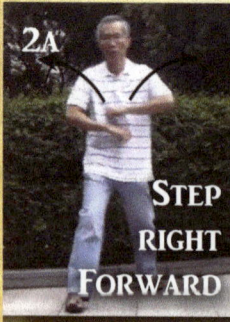

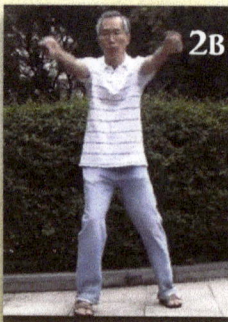

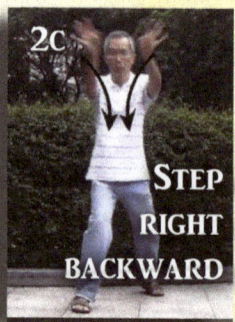

2A STEP RIGHT FORWARD

2B

2C STEP RIGHT BACKWARD

C **LINE ONE BEGINS** 2A - 8D →

execute basic skill #11 2A - 2F

ESSENCE OF 12 BASIC HANDS

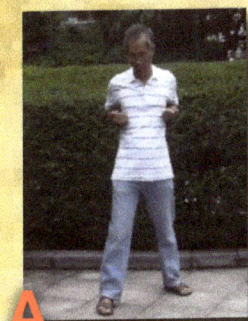

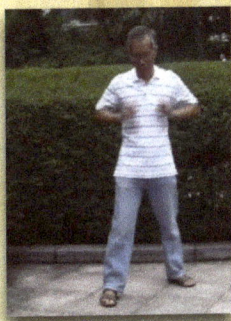

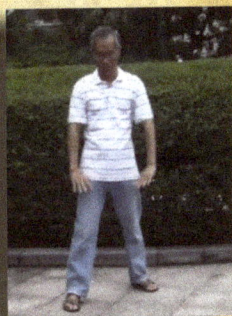

A →

raise the stomach - compress the ribs - round the back

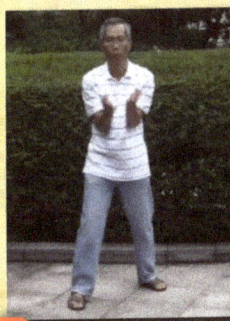

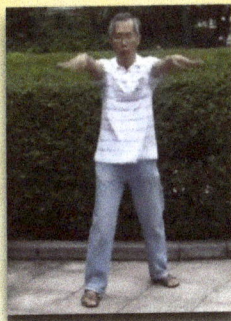

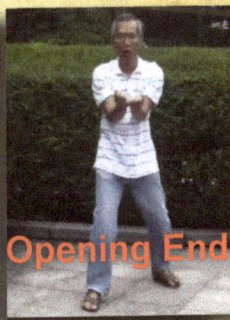

Opening End

B →

elbows inward - bil jee - gop shu

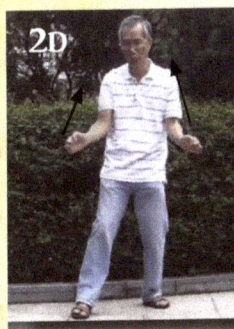

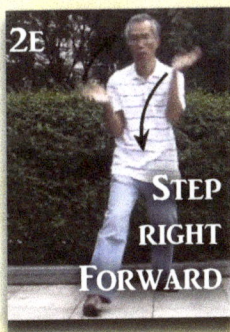

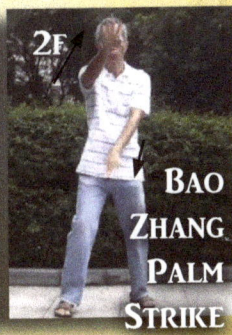

2D 2E 2F

STEP RIGHT FORWARD

BAO ZHANG PALM STRIKE

C →

basic hand skill #11: 2A - 2F

CHU KAI MING—2ND FORM

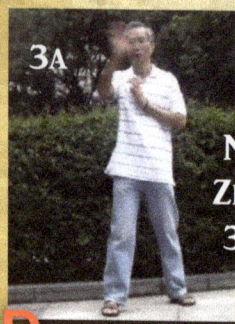

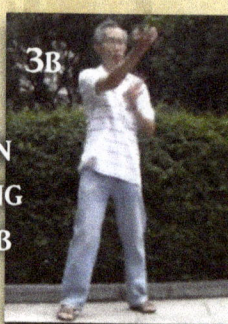

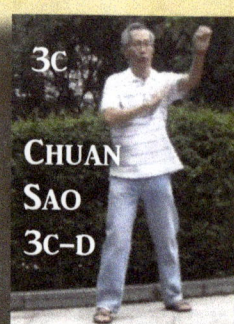

3A

3B

NIAN
ZHENG
3A-B

3C

CHUAN
SAO
3C-D

D

Basic Skill #3   3A - D

execute basic hand skill #3: 3A - 3D

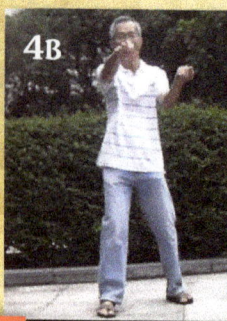

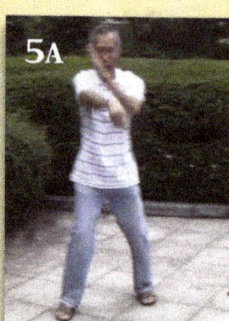

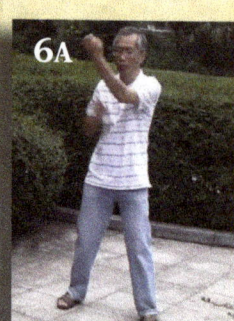

4B

5A

6A

E

Basic Skill #3 6A - B

execute basic skill #3 6A - B

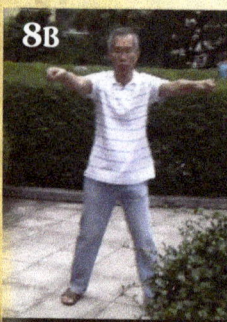

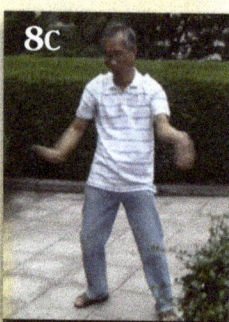

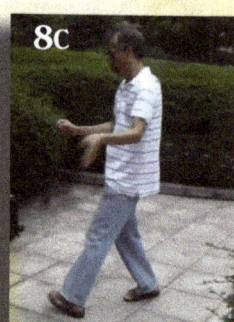

8B

8C

8C

F **Turn Around Sequence   8A - 8D**

each of the 4 lines turn around sequence repeats the same
with narp sao Locking Hands

ESSENCE OF 12 BASIC HANDS

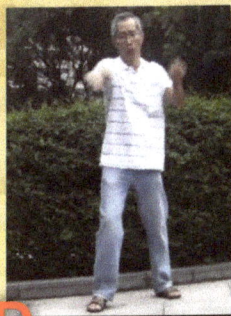

D →

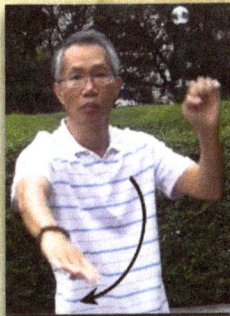

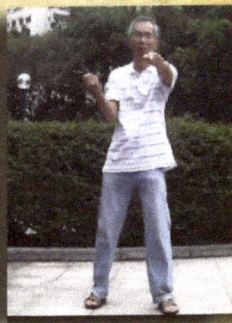

Basic Skill #4   4A - B →

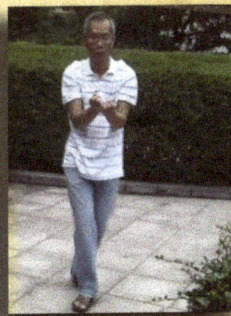

execute basic skill #4   4A - B

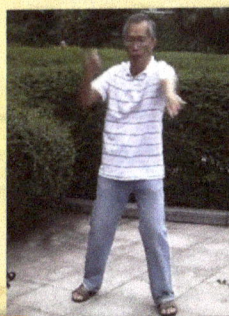

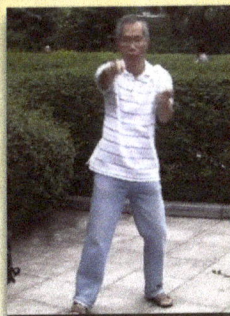

E →   **Basic Skill #4   7A**   **Turn Sequence** →

execute basic skill #4 - 7A;   begin turn around sequence

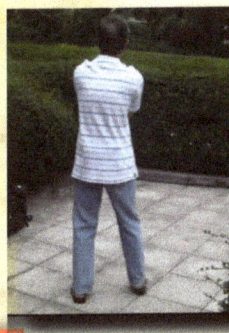

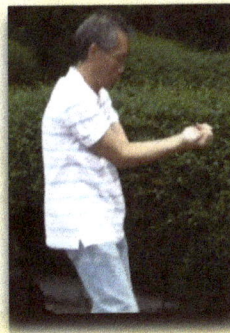

F →   **Turn Around Sequence   8A - 8D** →

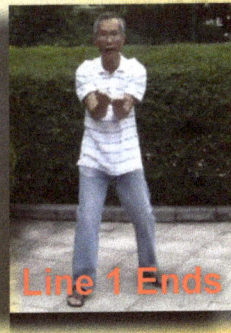

Line 1 Ends

8C-8D turn around in the opposite direction and gop shu

87

Chu Kai Ming—2nd Form

LINE TWO BEGINS 9A- 13D

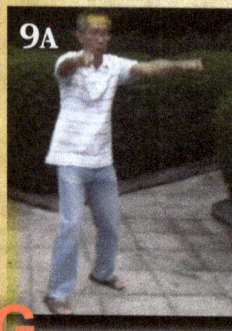

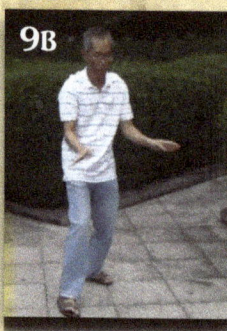

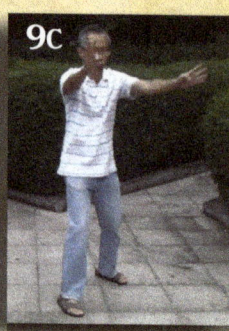

G →

line two begins, variation of basic hand skill #11: 9A-9C
(double bridge jek shu, gwak shu, bao zhang)

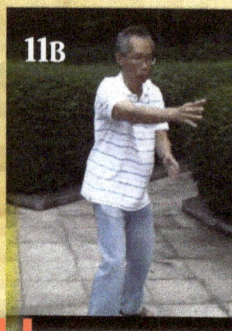

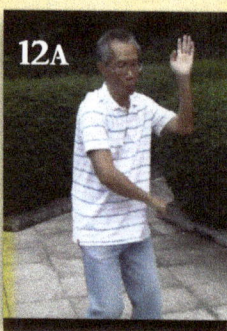

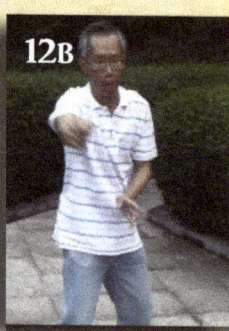

H →

left over hand trap and right outside gow choy 12A-12B

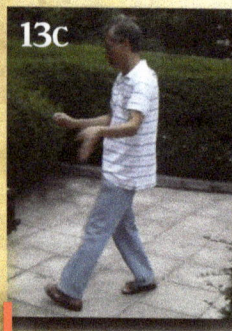

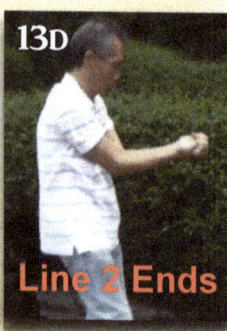

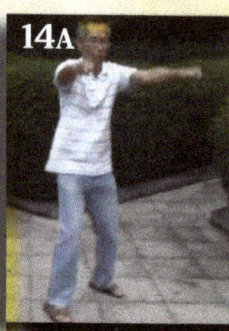

I →

LINE THREE BEGINS 14A - 18C

turn around in opposite direction and begin line three 13A - 13D

ESSENCE OF 12 BASIC HANDS

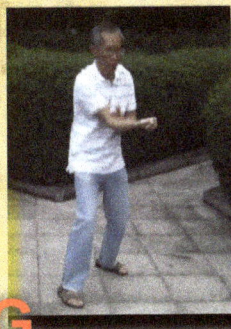

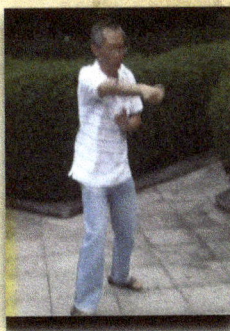

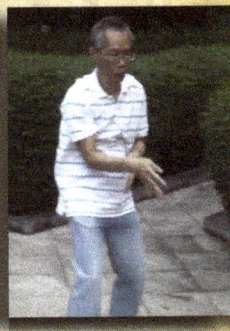

G

sink and gop shu single bridge - spit and right jek shu 10A-10B; sink and double bridge narp shu on centerline - spit and vertical bil jee centerline 11A-11B

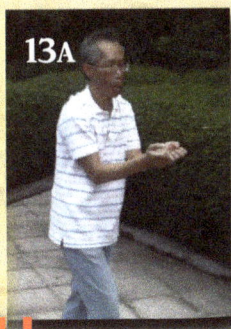

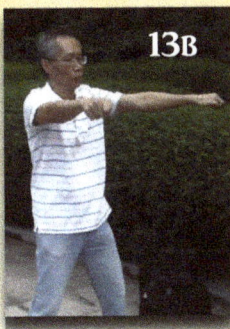

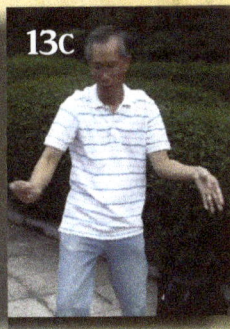

H

Turn Around Sequence   13A - 13D

cross step over & up to left horse; begin line two turn around sequence 13A - 13D

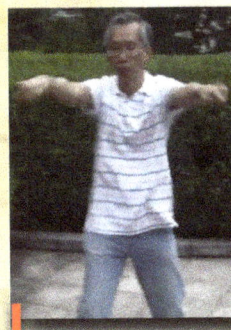

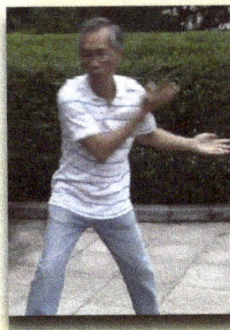

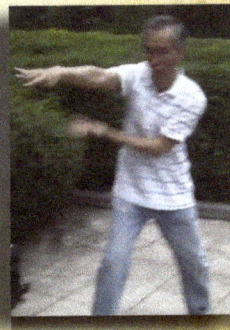

I

Basic Skill #7   14B - 15C

step right and double bridge jek shu; execute basic skill #7 14B - 15C

CHU KAI MING—2ND FORM

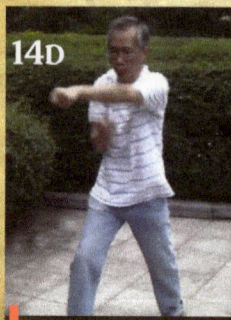

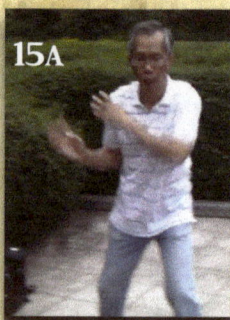

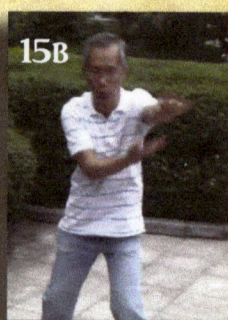

14D

15A

15B

J →

Basic Skill #7   14B - 15C

execute basic skill #7 14B - 15C

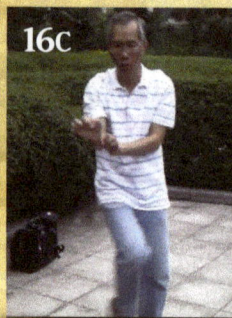

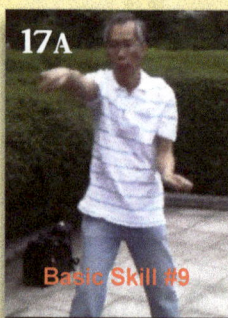

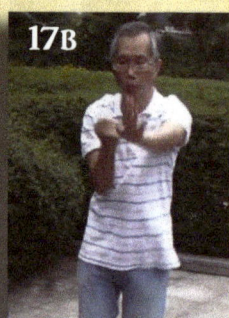

→

16C

17A

17B

K →

Basic Skill #9

→

execute basic skill #9: 17A; pull right lop shu and strike left bao zhang 17B

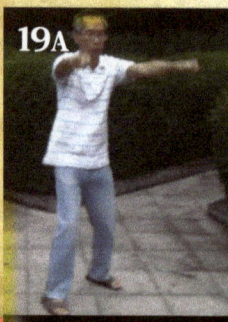

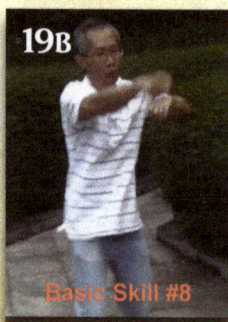

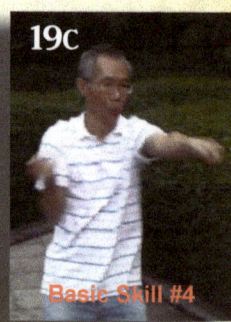

19A

19B

19C

Basic Skill #8

Basic Skill #4

L **LINE FOUR BEGINS** 19A - 21C:

→

step right double jek shu 19A; execute basic skill #8 - 19B; basic skill #4 - 19C

劉水第一代

ESSENCE OF 12 BASIC HANDS

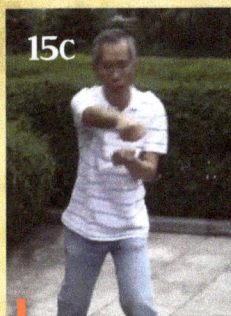

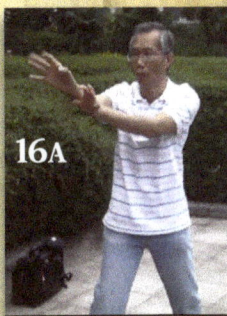

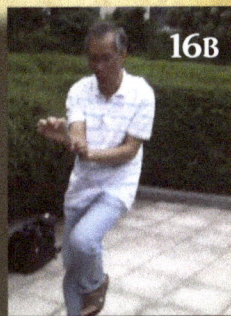

J

Qin Na Catch and Left-Right Chop Steps 16A - 16C

catch with claws and double knee strikes or deflections is common in hakka mantis

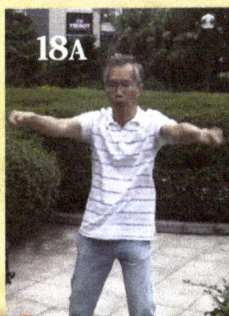

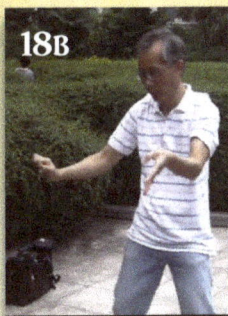

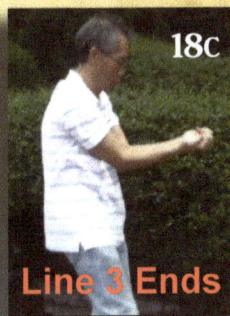

K

Turn Around Sequence 18A - 18C

begin line three turn around sequence 18A - 18C (repeat turn as in previous lines)

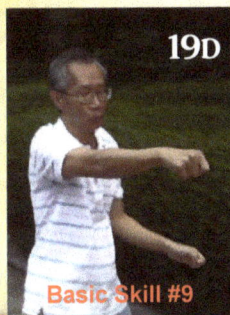

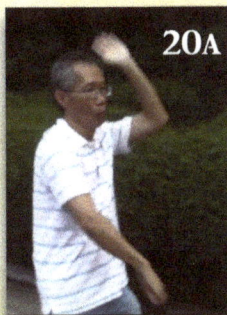

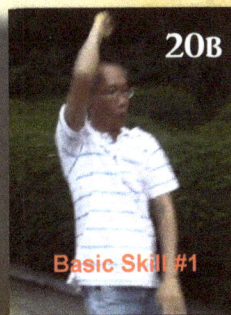

L

execute basic skill #9 - 14D; step forward trap left 20A and
big gow choy hammer fist 20B;

91

CHU KAI MING—2ND FORM

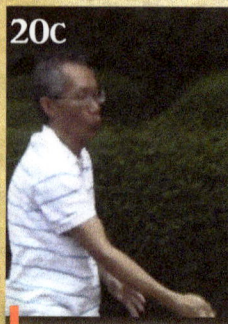

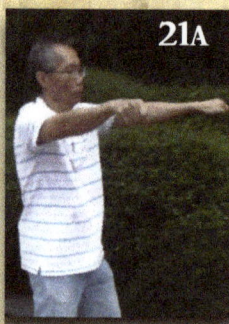

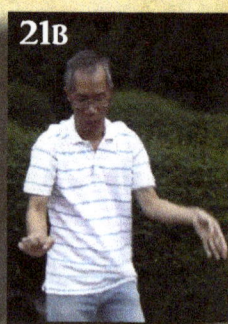

big gow choy splits centerline 20A - 20C; begin line 4 turn around 21A - 21C

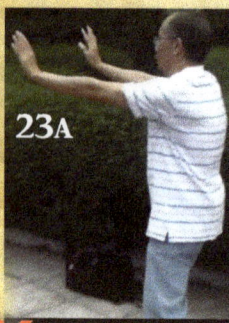

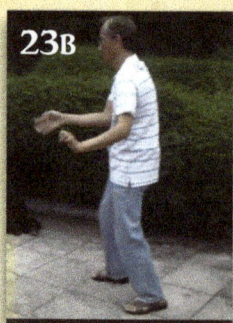

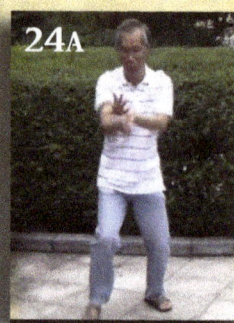

step (R) forward & double palm strikes 23A - 23B;   repeat a second time 23A - 23B

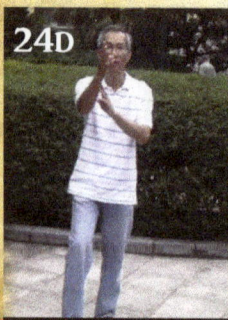

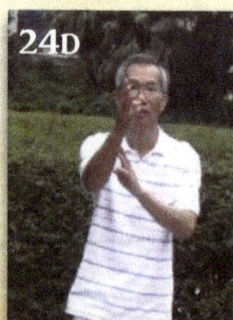

Although, Chan Sifu states his Sifu, Chu Kai Ming, did not have a salute, their forms do end the same as other first generation Lao Sui students (24A - 24D).

ending salute 24D

(single bridge 'hat yi sao' beggar's hand right - common to other Hakka styles also)

ESSENCE OF 12 BASIC HANDS

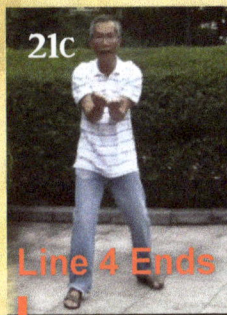
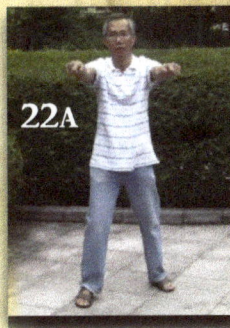
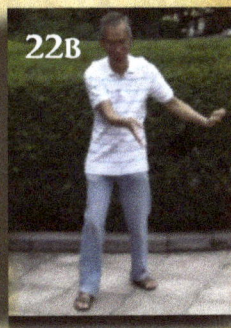

CLOSING SEQUENCE 22A - 24D:

step right & double jek shu 22A; step back with locking hand 22B

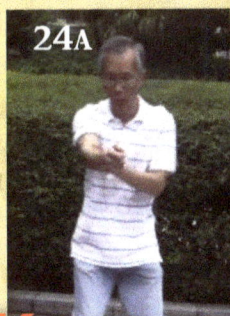
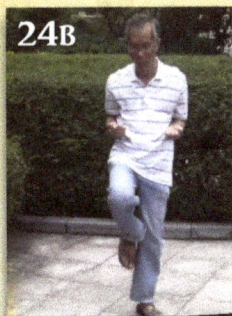
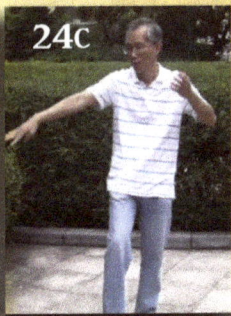

step (R) forward jik shu straight strike 24A - repeat a second time 24A
knee up elbows back 24B; strike pai shu side 24C

Three Principles of Mantis Form and Function

Relax, sink, and root, use feeling hand and turning power to strike the vital points—this is the summation of Mantis boxing. That is to say Mantis is based on a deep rooted horse, borrowing the opponent's force, and attacking his weak and vital points (root, feeling hand, vital points).

These brief boxing exhortations are contained within this Chu Kai Ming form. Understanding the principles will determine your ability in the training. Watch for the DVD of this form for further details. Read on now for interesting details of early Hakka Mantis.

Interviews with
Anthony Chan Sifu
Hong Kong, 2013

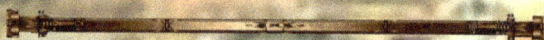

An Historian's
Perspective of
First Generation
Chu Gar Gao
From Lao Sui

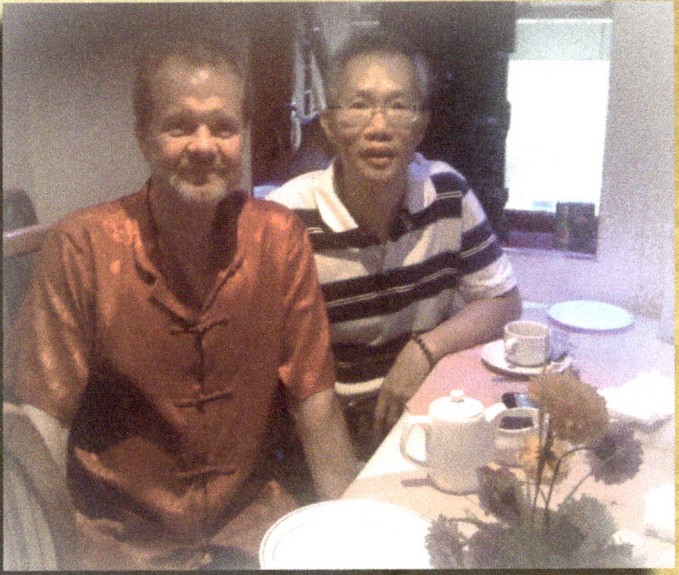

RDH (L), Anthony Chan (R), Hong Kong, 2013

Understanding and Ability
The Beginning and the End of Mantis

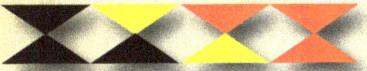

RDH: Up to this point, Chan Sifu, we've covered the complete transmission of single man training that your Sifu, Chu Kai Ming, received from Lao Sui, in the 1920-30s. Besides the Som Bo Gin closing sequence, what other differences were there from Sun Yu Hing's transmission?

AC: Sun Hing held a big party every year on his birthday and he always invited my Sifu and provided a big table for all of us. Sifu usually demonstrated Som Bo Gin and sometimes sparred with the students. If you have more photos of Sun Hing's annual birthday parties, you should look for Chu Sifu's picture. Sun Hing respected Chu and called him Sihing, older brother. As you said, my Sifu Chu was first generation Lao Sui and Sun, Chu Kwong Hua, Yip Sui and others were second generation.

AC: Sun Yu Hing had a very thick Hakka accent. I couldn't easily understand him. But in his transmission, he made the salute from the left side with left phoenix fist covered by right open hand, similar to Bak Mei.

RDH: Early on, circa 1980, in Mark Foon Sifu's Kwongsai Mantis school, he taught this but reversed and performed on the right side.

I saw you sometimes strike the double phoenix fists out and then bil jee spear fingers slowly and sometimes fast.

AC: My Sifu said to strike out closed fist, stop, and open the fingers rather slowly and when they feel full of blood, then stretch and round the back. But some people, also played the "three short power strike" quickly as in application and use. In both cases we close the fingers from "tiger's mouth", that is close the thumb and index fingers first, as if cracking a nut, and then each of the other fingers one by one while clasping the forearms in front of the body.

RDH: Where did your Sifu teach?

AC: In the Botanical Gardens, Victoria Park, Causeway Bay and a few other places. There weren't many students. Classes were held in the mornings from 7-8 am and afternoons 3-4 pm and evenings in Victoria Park. The tuition was 10 bucks a month back in those days and the same for everyone. However, if you were allowed to make a formal ceremony to become his disciple, you could give any amount.

RDH: What about Sun Yu Hing? Where did he teach?

AC: He opened a Chu Gar Mantis School in Tsuen Wan, New Territories. When I trained under Sun, in the early 1970s, there were little to no students. But, Tsuen Wan had a lot of martial arts schools at that time. Kwongsai Mantis was one of them. In 1973, there were still at least three Kwongsai Mantis Schools. Every year they had a big gathering with many schools and styles grouped together who put on a show and demonstrations to raise money for poor students.

RDH: And what years did your Sifu, Chu Kai Ming, teach in the park?

AC: I am not sure. Maybe as early as 1970. I started with him in 1972 until mid to late 1980s. But, in his latter days, he stopped teaching Chu Gar openly and only taught Tai Chi shadowboxing. He taught 80 something postures of the Yang Style.

I don't know what year Sun Yu Hing passed. I did not spend a lot of time with him because I already had a Sifu, Chu Kai Ming. And so, Sun Hing was very old fashioned and wouldn't accept me to learn from him formally.

RDH: So you only made ceremony to Chu Kai Ming?

AC: Yes, that was in 1972 or 73.

RDH: A lot of people nowadays especially, only use the hard bridge. But I see you also play the soft bridge. My Sifu Gene Chen, who you visited in USA, also played soft bridge. He said Chu Gar should be half hard, half soft.

I saw your opening sequence started a little differently.

AC: Yes, we had to put the hands, left on top of right, flat on top of the heart (center of chest). And then the whole sequence was breath control and we did it softly until the hands dart out with spear fingers - bil jee which was hard. This made Chu Sifu's teaching a bit different than some others.

RDH: So, what have you done in the time since your Sifu passed?

AC: Not much. Train myself. Once I posted on Google but then I deleted it! :) Sometimes Mantis seems under-appreciated in public forums. It is fate that you and I can meet in Hong Kong.

RDH: So after the warmups, Som Bo Gin form, 12 hands, Tan Zhuang Soft Bridge form, and Chu Sifu's last form, was there anything more?

AC: No, nothing. Even the weapons Chu Sifu didn't teach.

RDH: How about you personally? Did you train with others?

AC: Yes, many of the brothers who also trained Kwongsai Hakka Mantis. We trained together just like you and I are today. Just sharing and exchanging. Some closed their Jook Lum forms on the left salute like we talked about earlier.

RDH: What can you say about the Chu Gar breathing?

AC: It should be natural, inhale hands come in, exhale hands go out. Hold the breath when the hands go back to the waist chamber. But, Sifu said careful in this because if you get it wrong, it may cause you some internal injury.

RDH: How did you know Lam Pon Hing back then?

AC: Actually he is younger than I am. He should be still in Hong Kong these days and he used to work for the newspaper. He was a boxer, western boxer too. He learned Hakka Dragon style, Bak Mei, Mantis all from his father back in China. Because Hakka back then mixed all those Hakka Styles together. You know the Dragon is circular and the Bak Mei shoots straight forward.

I used to practice all this with Lam back in the early 1980s. We would train a couple times a week and I would keep extensive notes. But, I like Chu Gar Mantis more than the others. But, I also trained with Lam's Dragon Sifu as an outside gate student. Dragon used the right hand, right side salute like you said before.

Lam was my student. Today, now the Jook Lum and Chu Gar have many more forms than those days.

RDH: You are very skillful. I've watched you play half a dozen Hakka styles and as many forms now.

AC: Yes, I was Hakka Mantis and kungfu crazy! Just like you!

RDH: After your Sifu passed did you only train yourself or accept some students?

AC: Around 1992, I taught Yang style Taichi, Northern Mantis, and

Tiger and Crane, at a Hong Kong Youth Center.

RDH: Well, I'll share your Hakka boxing with others. Did your Sifu also train Shen Kung, the spirit boxing, or acupuncture, etc?

AC: He may have known that, but he didn't openly do it.

RDH: Well, how do you feel about the future?

AC: Not very optimistic. The tradition has changed. The forms have changed. Many are not following the original tradition today.

In the early days, teaching kungfu was not a profession. Kungfu masters were employed by a trade union or village to teach their members to protect themselves and defend against any rival gangs or villages. People learnt kungfu to protect themselves and the old masters taught one or two forms and mainly self defense techniques.

After 1970, a kungfu wave came and every street was full of kungfu schools. It gradually declined into forms performance and sport competitions. In the old days, a Hakka Master would teach you one form. Three good hands trained skillfully were better than 10 forms. Those days if a Sifu knew 四步惊劲 Four Gate, 標指, Bil Jee and 猛虎出林 Tiger leaving the Forest, he was a superman!

I treasure the simplicity of the old. Spending one's whole life to sharpen the weapon of self-defense purified the art more than showing a billion forms.

RDH: Did you meet Yip Sui Before?

AC: No, but I have brother-friends who were friendly with him. Chu Sifu said Yip changed the name. Yip was the last of Lao Sui's students at a time when Lao was sick several years before passing.

RDH: Did your Sifu mention Yang Shou and the Yang clan?

AC: Most of the time, Sifu talked about Tse Chung and Tam Wha. Tse Chung was my Sifu's training partner. Sifu said Tse Chung always stated if you knew Som Bo Gin and Dui Jong, then you already knew half of Chu Gar.

There were a number of those guys who were Lao Sui's first generation of students. And many who trained outside gate.

Liu Kwok Tung, the body guard of Dr. Sun Yat Sen, father of the Republic of China, Taiwan, knew 三步箭 Som Bo Gin. My Sifu also only knew 三步箭 Som Bo Gin and 散手 San Sao hand skills.

And 林生 Lam Sang, was well known. Those old guys who followed him in Hong Kong only learnt 三步箭 Som Bo Gin and 十八手 Eighteen Buddha Hands. I learned the 18 hands from an old guy, slightly different from yours.

Lao Sui taught 三步箭 Som Bo Gin, then 散手 San Sao basic hands, 对椿 Dui Jong 2 man, and 搓手 Chy Sao Grinding Hand. But as time changed, Yip Sui's school blossomed into many new forms.

If I was teaching now, I would teach 三步箭 Som Bo Gin, then 散手 San Sao basic hands, 对椿 Dui Jong 2 man, and 搓手 Chy Sao Grinding Hand. That is real kung fu, simple and effective. It is fighting art not performing art. But, this is just my opinion.

RDH: What say you about my Sifu Gene Chen's 1975 Chu Gar Certificate?

AC: Gene's Sifu, Dong Yat Long, was a student of Sun Hing and was very famous in Mantis circles. Sun Hing at that time was more famous than Chu Kwong Hua. There were many Chu Gar Gao factions in Hong Kong, and not only Lao Sui's lineage. In China, some places like 揭陽鴻江鄉 in Guangdong Province, are still practicing 朱家教 Chu Gar Gao, after five generations now. They did not adopt the Mantis name. They are different and their history is what Dong Yat Long said in the article you published for Gene Chen.

When I knew Dong Yat Long he was an herbalist and 跌打 Dit Da doctor. He opened a school in 慈雲山, Chi Yun Shan, a place full of Triad gangs. Dong's Sifu, Sun Hing, was in 荃湾二坡坊, Tsuen

Wan. His eldest son is a craftsman of copper and making iron tools.

In the USA, there is also a Chu Gar group of Sammy Wong. I have never seen any Mantis similar to their Chu Gar. Their Som Bo Gin is a combination of hand techniques.

Only one thing is true, in the old days, 1920s and 30s, of those who know Chu Gar, 90% only knew 三步箭 Som Bo Gin and 四門散手 Four Gate.

RDH: What years did your Sifu learn from Lao Sui?

AC: Well, he was a first generation student in Sau Kei Wan, when Lao first began teaching. The second generation of Lao's students, in the 1930s were on the Kowloon side of Hong Kong.

You see, Lao Sui's first Chu Gar school was near your Sigong Lam Sang's Kwongsai Mantis school in Sau Kei Wan. In the same area. I don't know if Lao and Lam Sang were friendly.

Also, there was another Jook Lum Sifu who operated a School. His name was Chung Sui. I think he was related to Chung Yel Chong, in China. Three Hakka Mantis Sifu in Sau Kei Wan then.

RDH: I have visited Chung Sui's student, Lam Hau Kit, in Sau Kei Wan. He is very skillful.

AC: Sau Kei Wan is a small area. There was another area, Yau Ma Di, where Lao Sui and the group always went to a restaurant. There was a rumor that he got into a fight over there and that is why he took sick and eventually died young.

The book said he was hurt by some wanderer who didn't appear very strong. And so Lao Sui kind of ignored him. But later suffered and got sick. Something like that.

This is all in that book we mentioned by Wong. But in those days, you couldn't talk about that with our Chu Gar Pai. Sifu would hit you on the head if you said such as this! But, it was written in a published book back then.

You see, I didn't even know my Sifu was Lao Sui's student until I made ceremony with him. It was only then he mentioned his Sifu was Lao and then talked a little about the other seniors and Pai.

RDH: Did you hear other stories about Lam Sang and his Jook Lum back then in Sau Kei Wan?

AC: Not really, but I believe he should have learned all of Chung Yel Chong's Mantis. But, I don't know why later they distanced themselves. It is just my opinion. When I compare all the old forms of Chu Gar, Jook Lum, and Lam Sang, then the Som Bo Gin of Lam Sang has all the elements of Chu Gar.

We talked about the Chu Gar summary of external and internal work earlier. Lam Sang's Jook Lum Som Bo Gin has already got all of this included. And he was practical because he taught those merchant marine seaman. They couldn't follow him ten years so they had to be practical. In order to survive he put the internal and external together with some Loose hands - San Sau. We didn't have that in Hong Kong at that time.

My Sifu knew one of those early Kwongsai students, surnamed Jie, in Sau Kei Wan but later on that guy went back to China and disappeared. I was too young when Sifu told me all this. I was not old enough to appreciate the history. I just wanted to learn the boxing and San Sao so I could fight!

Before WWII, they were building the Hong Kong old airport. And so a lot of Hakka people went to the Kowloon side to find work. Lao Sui and his second generation moved to Hong Hom over there. And because of the Hakka concentration of people, there were a lot of martial art schools opened.

The first issue of Real Kungfu magazine, back in the 1970s Hong Kong, should have featured my Sifu, Chu Kai Ming. However, it was changed to a Choy Li Fut Sifu because Sifu refused to wear the Kungfu suit. He just preferred his street clothes.

Later, the boss of New Martial Hero Magazine asked me to write an article about Chu Sifu. But, when I told this to Sifu he just dismissed the idea and said don't get mixed up with those guys! Sifu was very old fashioned.

The magazine boss asked me to come over and be a regular contributing editor because I could read and write English and Chinese. But Chu Sifu didn't allow me to do that. Sometimes, I think I lost a good chance to be a kungfu reporter!

RDH: Ha! Sometimes the old way is not always the best way! Perhaps, in this case, we can say that.

So, you were saying the author of that book about Chung Yel Chong, was not the Mountain Man pen name?

AC: There were two authors who used that name "Shan Ren" - Mountain Man. One was "Wo Shi Shan Ren - I Am A Mountain Man", the other was "Lian Fu Shan Ren - Buddhist Mountain Man". It was the latter who wrote that book about Southern Mantis Kungfu, in the 1950s.

RDH: So that book had step by step notes about Hakka Mantis? I only have a partial copy. Circa 1989, Yip Sui gave me Lee Kwun, his son-in-law's address, in New York Chinatown. Lee ran a bookshop and I went with Lam Sang's first geneartion, Wong, Eng, and Sun, to get a copy. But it wasn't available. Lam had that book but it had disappeared.

AC: It told that the secret of Kwongsai Mantis was "Yu Kiu" - left and right diagonal maneuvers. No pictures just all text. Exactly the hand written notes of Chung Yel Chong, step by step. And even so, it was so cryptic and esoteric that you could not understand exactly what was the meaning! Very hard to catch the meaning. It was the only book about Southern Mantis, at that time. And you can't find it anywhere today.

There was one old timer in Wanchai, a long time ago, that kept a lot of those old martial books and reprinted some. If he is still around, he may have it. During those days, there were many stories of famous Hong Kong Sifu, but only one written about Chung Yel Chong and Southern Mantis.

AC: There was only one article written about Lao Sui and that was in the Northern Mantis book by Wong Hon Fan. There used to be one copy of this book in the City Hall Library. I saw in the USA once, a complete catalog of Wong's writings.

RDH: Well, if we are speaking of the story of Lao Sui being hurt in Hong Kong, we must consider it contentious, since Wong was Northern and Lao Sui was Southern Mantis.

AC: Yes, and I don't believe the story because, at that time, Lao Sui ruled that area, and there was no way anyone could just walk up and approach him. He had many men always around him. It was the only place he went, and it was their Association's property and he was the leader. No one would dare to walk up on him because you wouldn't be able to get out, be able to get away, if you made trouble in their place!

That is one reason, I never mixed up much with the brothers (hing-dai) of Chu Gar Gao way back then. Because, some or many of them were gangsters. It was before the Triads were outlawed!

RDH: OK, Chan Sifu the recorder battery is going dead. We'll have to cut off here today and pick up again soon. Thank you for your brother-friendship and your Hakka Mantis transmission.

AC: Thank you! I hope others will benefit and appreciate the old tradition of Chu Gar too.

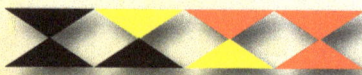

RDH NOTE: Any mistakes in translations, additions, or omissions to this book are mine alone and should not be attributed to Anthony Chan Sifu.

Advanced Two Man Forms

Be sure to review and study the Prerequisites as shown on page xii. Remember, a boxing maxim states, "Three years a small success, ten years a big success." The eight two man forms below comprise a two man long form that should be trained continuously and uninterrupted until one has achieved a "big success." Each form is only 1/8 of the method, although each is a stand alone form.

When you are skillful at each of the eight sets and can play them as one long form continuously, that is Advanced Two Man training. They must conform to the principles and fundamentals and include target practice to the vital points.

The Advanced Two Man Sets 11-18, must be trained by both people on both sides A and B. Only then have you completed one long form. It is likely to take 20 minutes or more, depending on your speed.

Advanced Two Man Forms — Year Two and Three

DVD Available by request. Prerequisite Volumes 1–10 (page xii).

- **Volume 11: Loose Hands One**

- **Volume 12: Som Bo Gin**

- **Volume 13: Second Loose Hands**

- **Volume 14: 108 Subset**

- **Volume 15: Um Hon One**

- **Volume 16: Um Hon Two**

- **Volume 17: Mui Fa Plum Flower**

- **Volume 18: Eighteen Buddha Hands**

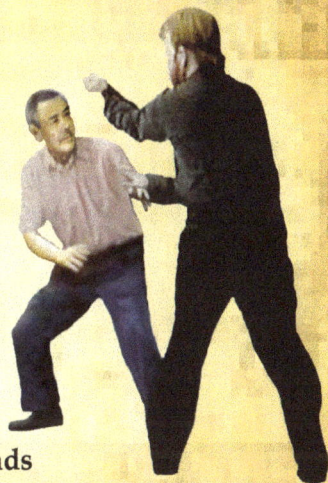

The long form sequence is one man plays the A side only of Loose Hands One (Volume 11) through Eighteen Buddha Hands (Volume 18) while one man plays the B side only. Without stopping, the two people switch sides and complete the forms (11-18) on both sides. A-B switch B-A is one long form. It is a pleasant feeling to complete the long form in training and leads to mastery of Hakka Mantis boxing.

CHINA HAKKA MANTIS HISTORY

Monk Som Dot's two disciples transmit
three Orders of Shaolin Praying Mantis Kungfu

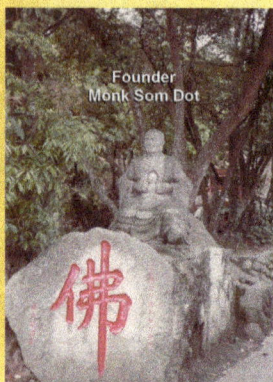

Founder
Monk Som Dot

It is said that Monk Som Dot was originally from Tibet and that he wandered extensively studying Shaolin boxing and medicine.

At the invitation of the Taoist Pope he travelled to Kwongsai Mt. Dragon Tiger and after settling there, he accepted two disciples, Wong Leng, an illiterate, but diligent disciple, and Lee Siem. Lee Siem later became known as Siem Yuen, which means capable of grasping the depth of Buddhism. And Wong Leng became known as Wong Do Yuen, capable in Taoism.

After some years, Som Dot sent his two disciples down the mountain to spread his art of Shaolin, which was divided into three orders. The first order taught the principle of 10 soft and one hard, and was taught only on the top of the mountain. The second order was half hard, half soft power. The third order was based on extremely forceful techniques. This is the reason the art is sometimes called a "three door or gate" art today.

In doing so, as they descended the mountain, Wong Do Yuen and Lee Siem Yuen, at the middle gate of the mountain, accepted a student named Chu Long Bot. Hiding the kungfu of the first order, they taught Chu Long Bot only the second order kungfu of Som Dot. At that time, the first order kungfu of Som Dot was not taught.

After learning the art, Chu, having no knowledge of the first order kungfu, betrayed Wong and Lee and used only the Chu surname to pass on what became 'Chu Gar Gao' - Chu Family Creed. The name was later changed again to "Chu Gar Praying Mantis" in Hong Kong.

Chu Long Bot later taught Chu An Nam, who taught Yang Sao and Lao Sui, who was a friend of Chu Kwei, who was the father of Chu Kwong Hua in contemporary times. This order of kungfu was originally taught only at the middle gate of the mountain.

Later, as Wong Do Yuen and Lee Siem Yuen went back down the mountain, at the lower gate, a praying mantis insect popped out in front of them. Wong, being the first to step off the mountain, proclaimed the mantis must be a sign from Heaven and to avoid further persecution of Som Dot's Shaolin teaching, the Shaolin art of three orders should simply be called Praying Mantis.

At the bottom of the mountain, a man surnamed Choy and nicknamed Tit Ngau, or Iron Ox, pleaded with sincerity to learn their kungfu and the two of them taught him Som Dot's third order of kungfu based on extremely forceful techniques.

Not knowing what to call the art, Choy, having no knowledge of the first or second order of Som Dot, eventually did the same as the Chu Clan and called the art Tit Ngau, or Iron Ox. Later a fellow named Chung Lo Ku learned from Choy and passed on this teaching as Chung Gar Gao in the East River region. This kungfu of the third order was taught at the bottom of the mountain.

In China, it is said each of Som Dot's three orders of Shaolin Kungfu has its advantage and each is worthwhile to learn and study.

Author's note: For an in-depth look at the origins and history of Southern Praying Mantis in China refer to the book, *Pingshan Mantis Celebration,* from SouthernMantisPress.com. Also, refer to the five volume eBook, *China Southern Praying Mantis Kung Survey*™ at chinamantis.com. (Monk Images are representations only; Som Dot left and Lee Siem above.)

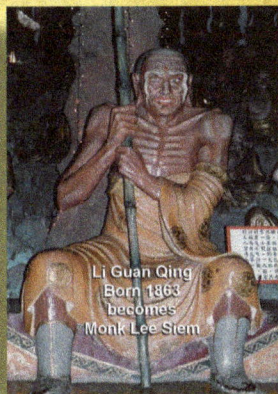

Note on Hand Names and Translations
In China, everyone has their own "jia xiang hua", or village dialect. Hakka is one such dialect and each clan or town may even have their own pronunciation of Hakka language. The names given herein are the names that are commonly used so that everyone is on the same page and understands which skill or hand is being talked about. It is less important what you call the skills, and more important that everyone understands.

The Chinese romanization herein is the same—it is written phonetically or what is common, so that it can be easily understood. Chinese names herein are not correct pinyin, purposely.

"Shu, Sao, and Shou" all simply mean "hand" and are often used interchangeably. Remember, once the stance, root and feeling hand is skilled, the whole body is one "hand".

About Southern Mantis on the Internet
The internet and DVDs can be a great aid to learning. How much better are DVDs than secretly peeking through holes in a fence or wall to learn Mantis? In the early days, sneaking a peek through a hole was quite common.

Nothing can replace the spirit and hand of a skillful teacher. But, the new media and resources are still a valuable asset. The internet, however, is also a large source of disinformation. Repeating what someone else said erroneously often becomes accepted as SPM "truth" without verification. There is a great deal of "false" information on the internet about Southern Praying Mantis.

An example is the 'Blanco' article. Circa mid 1990s, Blanco, from Hong Kong, called my office in the USA asking how to contact Southern Mantis teachers in China. I did not provide him any information. Southern Mantis teachers usually frown on unannounced visits from strangers. Later, he "compiled" his article using sources, such as my published works, without permission.

Much of his article is erroneous and needs correction. I encourage you to seek the truth for yourself. Do not follow any one blindly. Search and prove all things. The further you go downstream the murkier the water. Drink close to the source.

About the Photographs in this Book
The images are from my personal library. They were not made in a studio for glamor, but made on the spot with the various Teachers herein. Appreciate the images for what they are - natural shots of Sifu, in their own elements. None of the images can be made again—those days are gone. Sadly, many of the elder teachers have passed away, as well.

A Final Note

If you are interested in Southern Praying Mantis boxing, then I encourage you to read all of my books. They are genuine books of the true heritage of Southern Mantis. And although they are written by me, I can't really call them mine. I am just a transmitter of the heritage.

The branches of Southern Praying Mantis are from one root. Each has its advantage and is worthy of study. Although, I am first, Kwongsai Jook Lum Temple Mantis, and second, Chu Gar Mantis, both by Ceremony and Transmission, I am not biased or preferential. They are harmonious and may be taught side by side. The only difference is the depth of the transmission one receives.

Email me if you have a question, suggestion, or specific topic of Southern Praying Mantis you'd like addressed.

If you are interested in training by DVD or coming to Hong Kong or China to study Southern Mantis, then you may email me directly. I have a class in Guangdong, China, Cheng Chiu Sifu, teaches Chu Gar and Hakka Unicorn culture in Hong Kong and Wong Yu Hua Sifu's Guang Wu Tang is open. Welcome!

Roger D. Hagood
Standing Chairman
Bamboo Temple Chinese Benevolent Association, USA
Hong Kong Chu Gar Tonglong Martial Art Association
rdh@chinamantis.com

Vol 1: Pingshan Mantis Celebration Hardcover or eBook

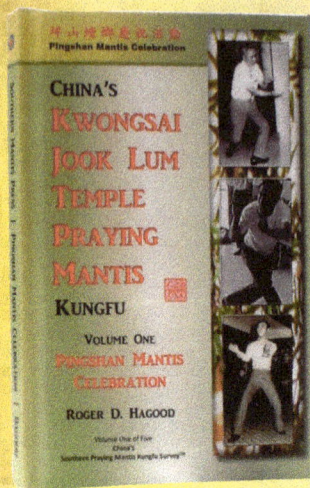

Pingshan Mantis Celebration

A rare book of China's Kwongsai Jook Lum Temple Praying Mantis Kungfu and Unicorn Culture.

Included are: Origins, history and practices of China's Kwongsai Mantis, rare and exclusive historical photographs never published before, the hometown of Kwongsai Mantis-Pingshan Town, how Wong Yuk Kong came to learn Hakka Mantis, why Wong Sifu went "mad" after a spell was cast, why Hakka Mantis is divided into "three orders" and what they are, three Wong Brothers who inherited Kwongsai Mantis, what Kwongsai Mantis boxing was taught early on and now, what happened when Kwongsai Mantis and Chu Gar first met, Hakka Mantis descending the mountain on horseback in 1917, English and Chinese translation of how Master Chung blossomed Hakka Mantis in South China, Hakka Culture along the East River, extensive interviews with inheritor Wong Yu Hua about sensitive topics, rules and regulations of Wong Yuk Kong's Mantis School, a Hakka Feast in

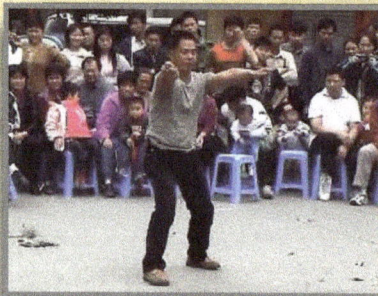

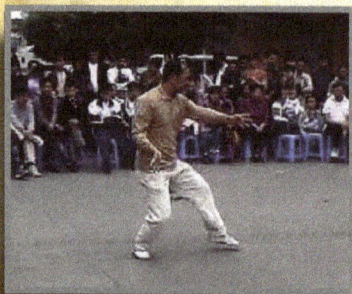

Pingshan Town, valuable Hakka Mantis resources online and off, Hakka Mantis boxing maxims and proverbs, dozens of Kwongsai Mantis boxing postures, staff, and sword pictures, rare never before published Jook Lum Mantis reliquary photographs, the Bamboo Forest Temple true heritage Dit Da liniment prescription and more.

Available at Amazon, Barnes and Noble, and other fine booksellers!
Search Keywords - Southern Mantis Press

Hardcover Collector's Edition Book

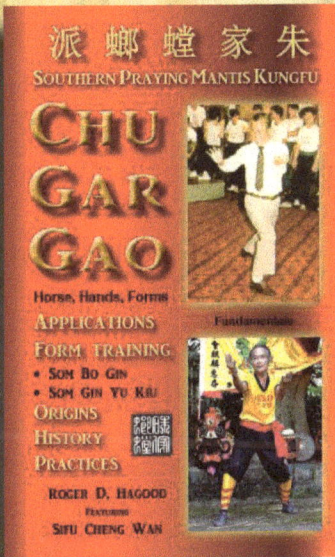

Chu Gar Gao: Southern Mantis

A rare treatise of Hakka Chu Gar Southern Praying Mantis boxing that includes: Chu Gar Mantis history, boxing transmission, six Chu Gar areas, three kinds of Chu Gar in China; Chu Gar Mantis personal records --- Sifu Chen Ching Hong, Sifu Yip Sui, Sifu Cheng Wan, Sifu Cheng Chiu, Sifu Dong Yat Long, Sifu Ma Jiuhua, Past Masters in Charge; Chu Gar applications --- Single Bridge Tsai Sao, Double Bridge Dui Jong, Mang Dan Sao Dui Jong, Ying Sao Shadow Hand, Gow Choy Hammer Fist, Locking Hands, Bridge, Tan Sao, and Ginger Fist, Double Bridge Gwak Sao, Sticky Hand and Intercepting Hand Bao Zhang Palms; Chu Gar shadowboxing forms in pictorial--Som Bo Gin (Three Step Arrow) and Som Gin Yu Kiu (Three Arrows Shaking Bridge form); and more.

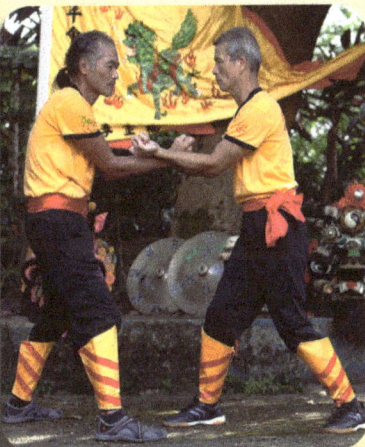

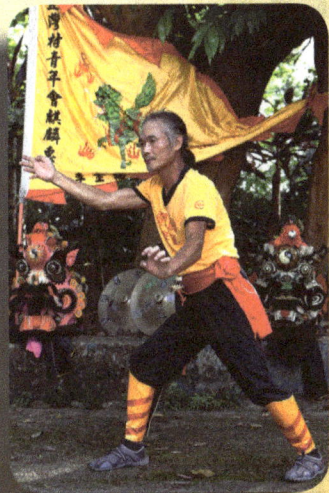

Available at Amazon, Barnes and Noble, and other fine booksellers!
Search Keywords - Southern Mantis Press

VOL 2, 3, 4: China Mantis Survey Hardcover or eBook

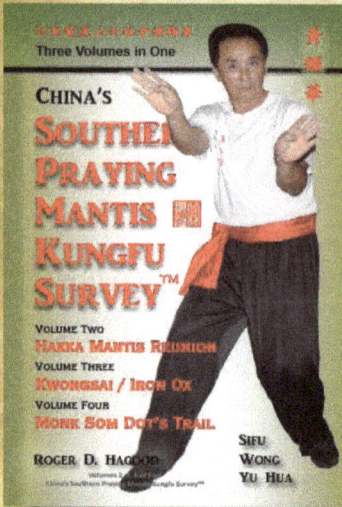

A rare three volume book of China's Hakka Kwongsai Jook Lum Temple and Iron Ox Praying Mantis boxing.

V olume Two, China Hakka Mantis Reunion, includes: Three Orders of Som Dot's Shaolin Mantis revisited, Hakka Mantis blossoms in Huizhou, Elder Lok Wei Ping-a Chu Gar and Kwongsai Sifu, Chung Yel Chong teaches one form, Kwongsai and Chu Gar clash in the 40s, Sifu Wong Gok Hong takes the lion head away, Lau Say Kay Sifu plays non-standard Kwongsai Mantis, Sifu Lai Wei Keung first Instructor in 1948, One Kwongsai form originally taught, Two methods of beggar hands, Sifu Cho Gum, Sifu Wong Yu Hua, Fairy hands cause a slap on the rear, Lok Sifu plays 34 Plum Blossom Staff, All Mantis is one family, Lai Sifu plays 34 Plum Blossom staff and more!

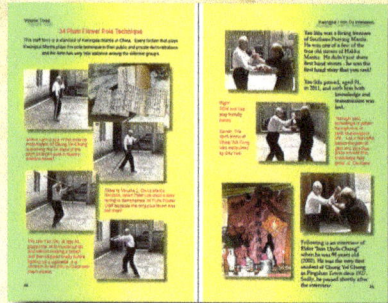

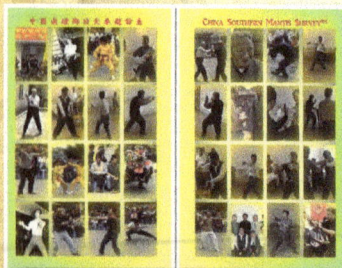

V olume Three, Kwongsai / Iron Ox Interviews, includes: Records of the elders and knowledge lost, Sifu Yao Kam Fat, Wong Yuk Kong opens Kwongsai Mantis in Hong Kong, Wong Yuk Kong visits Lao Sui's Chu Gar school, Wong Yuk Kong defeats 10 assailants, Yao Sifu plays three steps-three scisscors old form, Similarities in Hakka Mantis, Yao Sifu plays 34 Plum Blossom staff, Spirit Shrine of Wong Yuk Kong, Elder Sifu Chung Wu Xing first disciple

VOL 2, 3, 4: Three Volumes in One Hardcover Book

of Chung Yel Chong, Iron Uncle Chung friend of Lam Sang, Iron Uncle Chung smokes opium with Lam Sang and Master Chung in the 1930s, Sifu Yang Gun Ming student of Chung Yel Chong, Dit Da Doctors by lineage, Hakka Mantis prohibited in the Cultural Revolution, Sifu Xu Men Fei Iron Ox Hakka Mantis, Iron Ox taught only 2 months a year, Xu Sifu plays Iron Ox Second Door form-Red Flag Staff-and Third Door form, Iron Ox challenges Wong Yuk Kong's Kwongsai Mantis, Iron Ox Secret Drill Hand not taught, and more.

Note: The hardcover book has supplemental information not contained in the eBook.

Volume Four, On Monk Som Dot's Trail / Chung Yel Chong Family Interviews, includes: Sifu Chung Wei Fei grandson of Master Chung, Master Chung Yel Chong as a boy accepted by Monk Lee, Chung Go Wah son of third ancestor Master Chung, Master Chung's boxing and Dit Da Medicine books, Third Ancestor Chung teaches Kwongsai Mantis in Hong Kong 1920s, Master Chung kills a man in self-defense, Master Chung's three generations under one roof, Sifu Lee Kok Leung outlines his Kwongsai Mantis teaching, Sifu Patrick Lee plays Mantis in Pingshan Town, Lee Sifu's History of Kwongsai Mantis, On Som Dot's Trail - Shanxi Jook Lum Temple, Oldest of the Temple Halls, Chung and Monk Lee return South six months on horseback, Kwongsai Dragon Tiger Mountain of Shaolin boxing and spiritualism, The bottom line about Kwongsai Jook Lum Temple, Lam Sang's Kwongsai spiritualism and amulet, Monk Lee Siem looks like a ghost, Jook Lum Temple in Hong Kong, Jook Lum Temple in Macau, Map of Jook Lum Temples in China with Hakka Mantis boxing, Abridged China Hakka Mantis history, Guang Wu Tang Martial Hall of Wong Yuk Kong in 2012, Mission statement of Guang Wu Tang Kwongsai Mantis, Sifu Wong Yu Hua in 2012, Miscellanies, Resources, Train in China. Kwongsai Mantis and Iron Ox boxing and staff forms in sequence, and more.

- Hardcover
- Full color
- 330+ photographs
- 128 pages

Available at Amazon, Barnes and Noble, and other fine booksellers!
Search Keywords - Southern Mantis Press

Hardcover Collector's Edition Book

Eighteen Buddha Hands
Kwongsai Jook Lum Temple Mantis

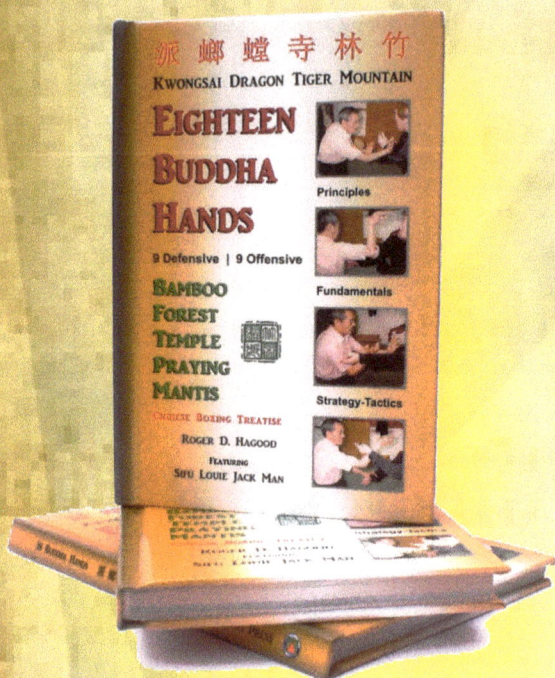

A rare instructional treatise of Chinese boxing from the Kwongsai Dragon-Tiger Mountain, Bamboo Forest Temple, Praying Mantis Clan, as transmitted by the late Grandmaster Lam Sang.

Details include stories of Lam Sang's supernatural ability such as Poison Snake Staff, Sun Gazing, and Light Body Skills. Boxing principles elaborated are Body posture, Rooting, Sinking, Center-line, Spiral power, Contact-control-strike, Intercepting and sticky hand, Bridging, Anticipating-telegraphing, Dead and live power, Form and function, 4 word secret, Dim Mak vital points and more.

Boxing Fundamentals included are Footwork: Chop, Circle, Advance, Shuffle step, Turnarounds, Side to side; Kicks, Sweeps, Takedowns, Grappling, Chin Na Seizing, Hook hands, Elbow strokes, Dui Jong, Sticky hands, Forms, and Phases of training. Eighteen Buddha Hand techniques, 9 defensive, 9 offensive, are illustrated in color with instruction in attributes, function and vital point targeting. Boxing maxims of strategy and tactics are included.

Available at Amazon, Barnes and Noble, and other fine booksellers!
Search Keywords - Southern Mantis Press

MantisFlix™ Video eBooks

60 Years of Southern Mantis Movies and Events!

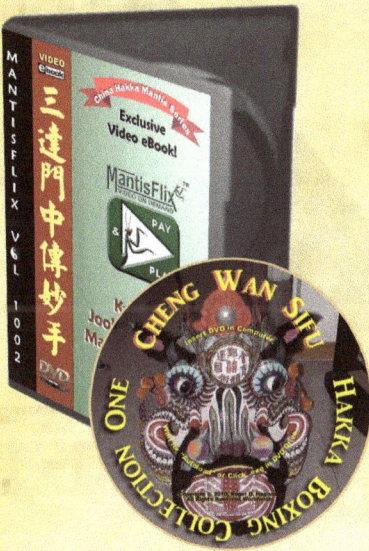

Wong Fei Hong and the Jook Lum Temple

Volume 1001 - Hong Kong 1954

B/W Classic Movie Exclusive! 100,000 plus clip previews on YouTube. Get your full copy now!

Kwongsai Mantis Celebration

Volume 1002 - Pingshan Town, Guangdong, China

Late Sifu Wong Yuk Kong Kwongsai Jook Lum Clan 35th Anniversary Celebration, circa 2003.

Hakka Boxing Collection One
Volume 1003 - A rare collection of Hakka Boxing.

Hakka Boxing Collection Two
Volume 1004 - A second rare collection of Hakka Boxing.

Chu Gar Cheng Wan Celebration
Volume 1005 - Join the 1989 Cheng Wan Chu Gar Mantis Celebration in Hong Kong! Cheng Wan Sifu was the inheritor of Chu Gar descended from Lao Sui.

View and Enjoy Video Previews Online:
www.MantisFlix.com

Online

Our Family of Hakka Mantis Websites
Visit and Enjoy! Informational, Educational, Instructive

www.SouthernMantisPress.com

A ten year ongoing research in China
of the origins, history and practices of Southern Mantis!

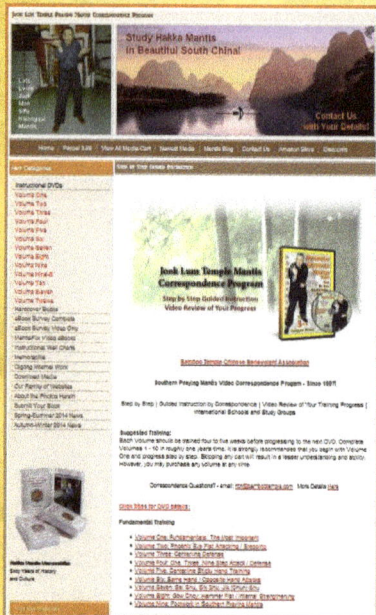

Dedicated to the late Wong Yuk
Kong Sifu in China!
chinamantis.com

The Bamboo Temple Association
is a mutual aid fraternity.Join
us and become a member,
School, Branch or Study Group
today!Dedicated to the late Lam
Sang Sifu's teaching in the USA.
bambootemple.com
bambootemple-chicago.com
btcba.com

These sites reveal many China
Kwongsai Mantis Sifu who have
heretofore remained silent about
the teaching of Kwongsai
Dragon Tiger Mountain Bamboo Forest Temple Mantis and
outlay the lineage of Hakka Mantis as stated in China.
kwongsaimantis.com
somdotmantis.com

This site details the complete history of Chu Gar Gao Hakka
Praying Mantis as descended from the late Lao Sui in Hong Kong
and Hui Yang (Wai Yearn), China.

Resources

(con't) Dedicated to the late Cheng Wan Sifu who passed in 2009.
chugarmantis.com

This site is dedicated to the late Xu Fat Chun Sifu and speaks of
the history of Iron Ox Hakka Praying Mantis in Pingdi Town,
Guangdong, China.
ironoxmantis.com

Historical Hakka Mantis Flix! Some 60+ years of Hakka Southern
Praying Mantis Kungfu movies and events in video eBooks!
mantisflix.com

Our dedicated South Mantis Tube. We have several hundreds of
hours of videos in our Hakka Mantis archives dating back to 1950
in China that we hope to share with you!Feel free to share.Upload
your Southern Mantis or Hakka video now!
southmantis.com

Genuine Internal Work - the original 11 month correspondence
course of Tien Tao Qigong.
tientaoqigong.com

Ancient Methods to achieve vitality and a healthier well-being! The
Oriental Secrets Series of Qigong.
oss.tientaoqigong.com

Visit our daily YouTube feed of only
Southern Praying Mantis videos!
chinamantis.com/youtube

And our YouTube channel:
youtube.com/chinamantissurvey

Southern Mantis Instructional Playing Cards

**Kwongsai Mantis
18 Buddha Hands**

Card Backs: Various Sifu of Lam Sang's generations in multiple postures

Card Fronts: Two man application photos, Text instruction, Instructive maxims

Includes the 18 Buddha Hands and more of Kwongsai Hakka Mantis

**Key Benefits
of our Card Decks**

- 54 Cards with Hakka Mantis
- Customized Front and Back
- Full Vibrant Color!
- Instructional
- Educational
- Informative
- Rare and Exclusive Content and Photographs
- Entertaining - Play Hakka Mantis Cards with your friends

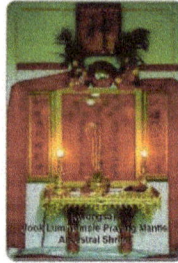
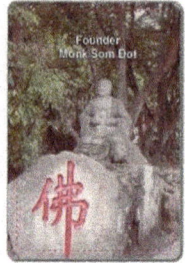
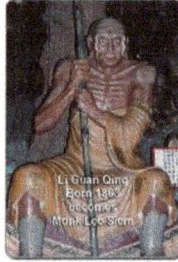
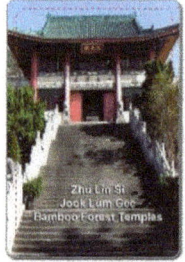
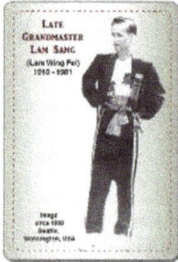
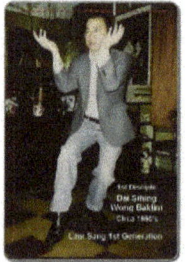
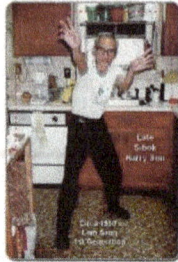
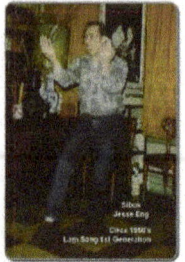

New Media from Southern Mantis Press.com

18 Buddha Hands—Instructional Card Deck

Card Deck Use Includes

- Useful gifts for martial artists
- Instructional and Informative
- Invaluable Heirloom of Hakka Mantis Masters

Card Decks Include

- 54 card deck in standard size
- Made from 100% casino quality card stock
- Clear plastic case included

Wholesale Inquiries Welcome

Other Decks Include:

- Chu Gar Mantis - "Fundamentals"
- China Kwongsai Mantis - "Celebration"

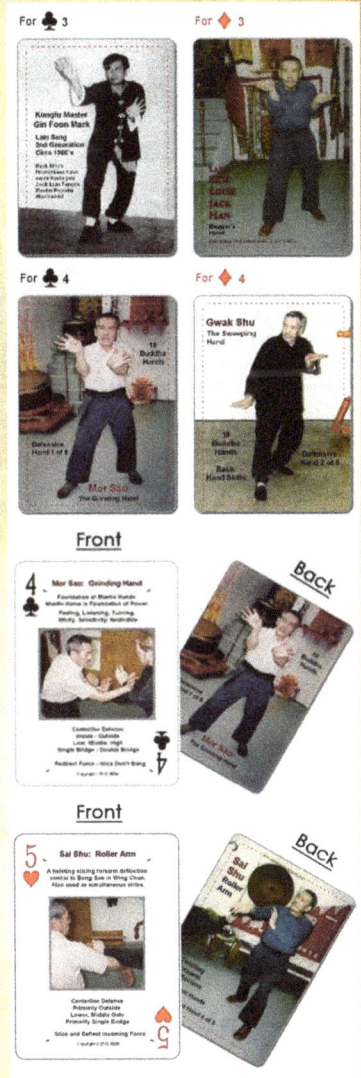

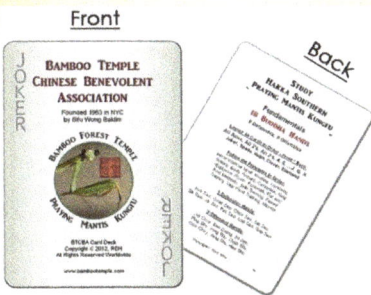

For order info email:

cards@chinamantis.com

Correspondence Program - Step by Step

Jook Lum Temple Mantis
Correspondece Program
in 18 Volumes
Video Review of Your Progress

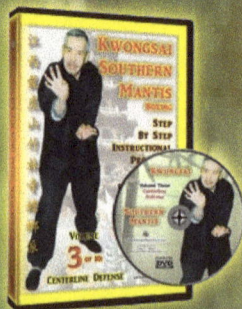

Year One Training
Volume One: Fundamentals; The Most Important
Volume Two: Phoenix Eye Fist Attacking / Stepping
Volume Three: Centerline Defense
Volume Four: One, Three & Nine Step Attack / Defense
Volume Five: Centerline Sticky Hand Training
Volume Six: Same Hand / Opposite Hand Attacks
Volume Seven: Sai Shu, Sik Shu, Jik (Chun) Shu
Volume Eight: Gow Choy; Hammer Fist-Internal Strength
Volume Nine: Footwork in Southern Praying Mantis
Volume 10 Chi Sao Sticky Hands and Passoffs

Advanced Two Man Forms — Year Two and Three
Available by request. Prerequisite Volumes 1– 10.
Volume 11: Loose Hands One
Volume 12: Som Bo Gin
Volume 13: Second Loose Hands
Volume 14: 108 Subset
Volume 15: Um Hon One
Volume 16: Um Hon Two
Volume 17: Mui Fa Plum Flower
Volume 18: Eighteen Buddha Hands
All 8 two man forms must be trained as one continuous set on both A - B sides.

Summary Year One
http://www.chinamantis.com/first-year-training.htm

Summary Year Three:
http://www.chinamantis.com/summary-of-training.htm

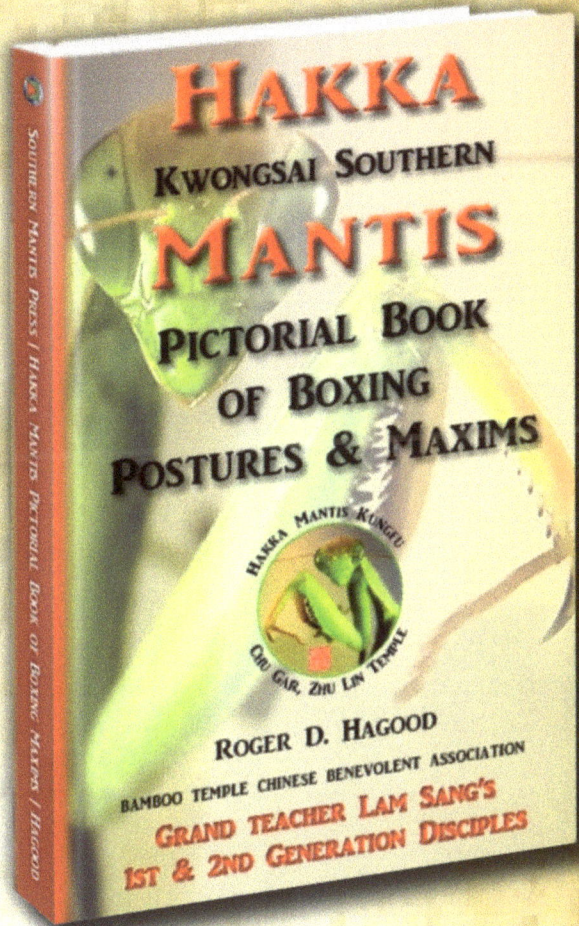

Welcome to visit the Author!

Your email correspondence is welcome and do visit and study Hakka Southern Praying Mantis with me in beautiful sunny south China!   I am an Author, Publisher and Producer of eBooks, books, journals, videos and 7 International martial arts newsstand magazines in 15 countries with 48 years in training and teaching martial arts and some 20+ years living in China and Asia!

Currently residing in beautiful sunny south China for the last 14 years where I teach Southern Praying Mantis.   Join my class in Guangdong today!

RDH
Pingshan Town
Summer 2015

More Bio:
http://www.chinamantis.com/roger-d.-hagood.htm
Email:
rdh@chinamantis.com

Study Hakka Mantis and Unicorn in China

Study in Beautiful South China!

Train Hakka Unicorn Culture at Guang Wu Tang - The Martial Hall of Wong Yuk Kong! Email your details for consideration today. rdh@chinamantis.com

SOM BO GIN SINGLE MAN

Three Step Arrow Form

Few Southern Mantis Clans have retained the "Tan Zhuang" Soft Power Som Bo Gin. In this form, the three steps forward each execute flicking the fingers out with soft "tan ging" power (A-C) instead of the common three arrow punching followed by finger tip strikes.

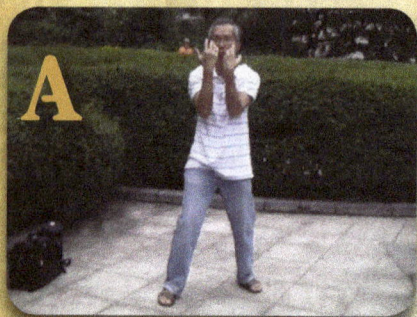

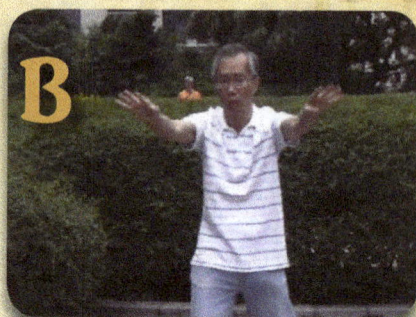

This "Som Bo Gin" form, in Southern Mantis, is written, in Chinese, by three different names: "Three Step Arrow" in Chu Gar, "Three Steps Forward" in Lam's USA Kwongsai Mantis, and "Three Steps Scissors" in China's Kwongsai Mantis.

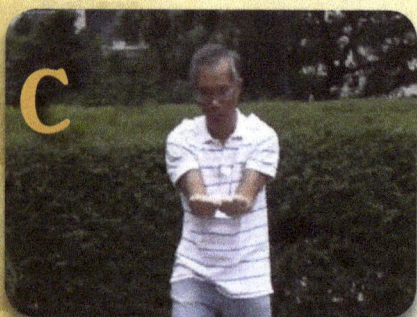

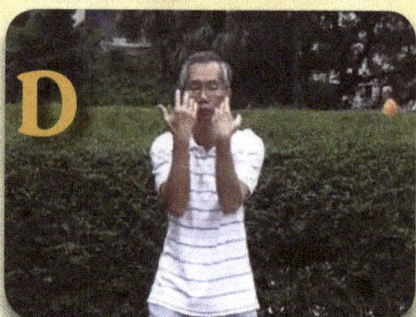

Read further, inside this book, about the form pictured here. And use the link below to garner detailed information about both Som Bo Gin Single Man and Two Man forms.

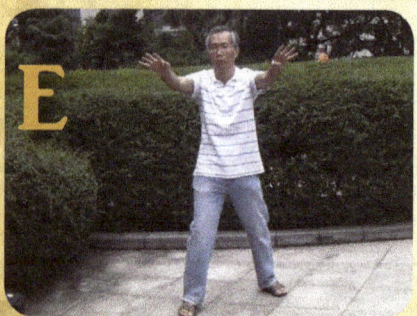

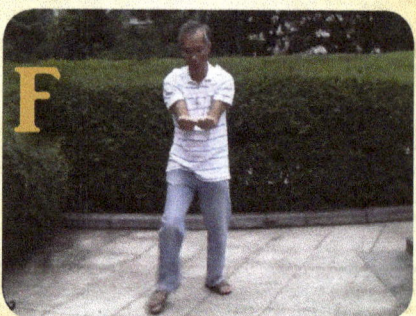

LINK TO SOM BO GIN TWO MAN FORM

southernmantispress.com/southern-praying-mantis-book-005.htm

三步進弹桩　SOFT BRIDGE

Refer to Page 70 for details.

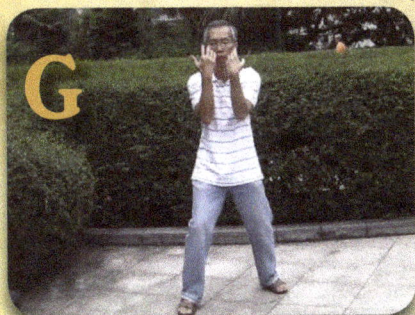

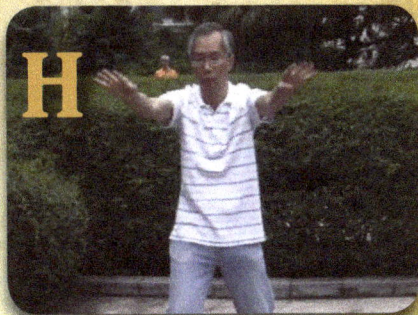

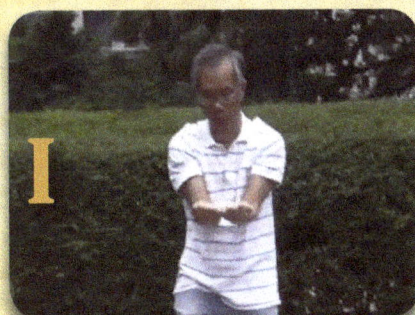

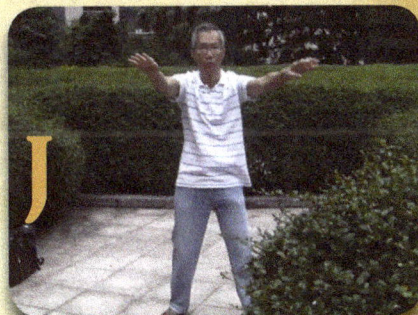

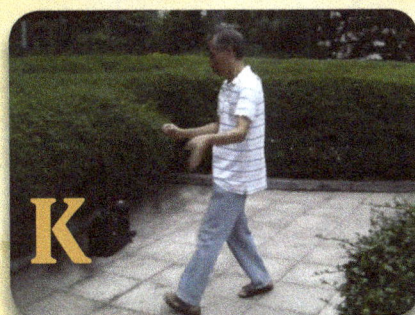

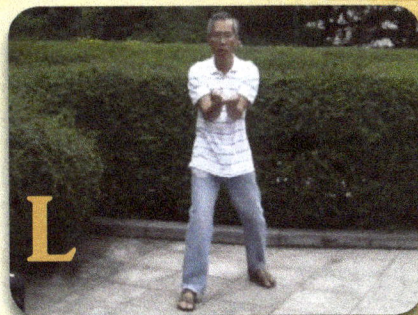

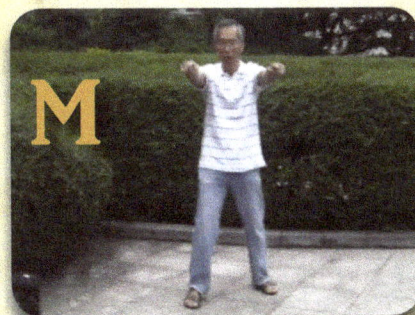

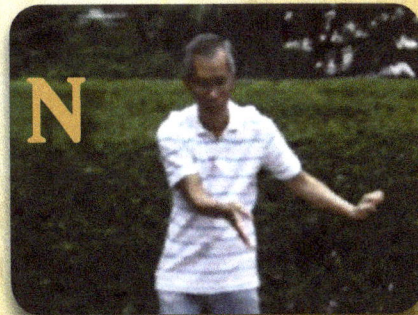